Creating Optimal Relationships

Creating Optimal Relationships

Use of the Voltage Concept with Couples

Kathryn Elliott and James Elliott

ROWMAN & LITTLEFIELD
Lanham • Boulder • New York • London

Published by Rowman & Littlefield
A wholly owned subsidiary of The Rowman & Littlefield Publishing Group, Inc.
4501 Forbes Boulevard, Suite 200, Lanham, Maryland 20706
www.rowman.com

Unit A, Whitacre Mews, 26–34 Stannary Street, London SE11 4AB, United Kingdom

British Library Cataloguing in Publication Information Available

Library of Congress Control Number: 2015949674
ISBN: 978-1-4422-3810-7 (cloth : alk. paper)
eISBN: 978-1-4422-3811-4

∞™ The paper used in this publication meets the minimum requirements of American National Standard for Information Sciences—Permanence of Paper for Printed Library Materials, ANSI/NISO Z39.48-1992.

Printed in the United States of America

Contents

Acknowledgments

Our creation of Anthetic Therapy has a long history dating back to the beginning of my (James) study of psychotherapy in 1947 when I read Karen Horney's books and learned the importance of "shoulds," basic anxiety, and the three personality styles: compliant, detached, and expansive. I became aware of the superego from reading Freud but was made conscious of its destructiveness from Edmund Bergler's books. I became conscious of "parts" from Eric Berne's Transactional Analysis seminars. From Steward Shapiro and Fritz Perls, I learned about empty chair work. From an article by Louis Paul, I got the idea that empty chair work could be used to disarm the Inner Critic. I modified it considerably and named it Anthetic Dialogue. From the work of Albert Ellis, Aaron T. Beck, and other Cognitive-Behavioral Therapists, I integrated many insights. From the work of Alfred Adler, I learned about compensation and modified it considerably in the Anthetic theory of compensation.

Anthetic Relationship Therapy had its inception in 1964 in my growth groups in Palo Alto, San Francisco, and Berkeley, California. It is to the participants in these groups, and to the couples who consulted us from 1989 to the present, that we owe so much gratitude. Their hunger for relationship happiness, along with their courage in exploring it, led to the creation of the High-Voltage Relationship (HVR) concept and skills.

I (Kathryn) also want to thank my graduate students for their wholehearted acceptance of these ideas and their participation in early research.

We want to acknowledge and offer our deepest gratitude to Dr. Eric Green for his love of us and his valuing of our work over the years and for opening the door to our sending it out into the world in this form.

Thank you to editors, Amy King and Alison Pavan, at Rowman & Littlefield, for seeing the value of the voltage approach to couple work and helping us articulate it for our colleagues.

For our team at Anthetic Therapy Center who love Anthetic Therapy and devote themselves to sharing it (Marianne Prejean, Tamra Griffin, Scott Mire, and Diane Dodt) our deepest gratitude. Thank you also for your support and love since Jim's death and for carrying on the work while I (Kathryn) have prepared this manuscript for publication. Thank you too to Linnette Abshire for her friendship and support to Jim and to me.

J.E. & K.E.

Introduction

> Inside you is a great reservoir of magical energies for loving in a deep way, even in a mythic way.
>
> —*Hearts Entwined: The Love Letters of Therapist-Soulmates*

So ends the introduction to our book of love letters from the first six months of our relationship. It is a fitting quote to introduce this book which offers our model for intimate relationships. The philosophy contained in this quotation represents a culmination of our observations over the course of forty years of group and couple therapy. As we analyzed the greater than 50,000 two-person interactions observed during those sessions, we were compelled by an immense realization: Each individual has access within to an artesian well of love such that if blocks could be removed, a stream from that reservoir would flow optimally in his or her relationships.

Distilled from our observations was the identity of a primary block for the flow of that love. It was an internal entity called the Inner Critic, the influence of which in each person leads to most of the conflict, pain, and suffering entailed in relating to one another. In the earliest days, before we met, James experimented with ways to help people become free from that influence. What emerged was more than a mere set of skills; instead was a whole new approach to working with individuals and couples, that is, Anthetic Therapy and Anthetic Relationship Therapy. It was a work that took James up in its grasp and became his life calling.

As his clinical practice and inquiry continued, he discovered the importance of inner figures in individual and couple functioning. With his background and interest in existential philosophy, Karen Horney's psychology, as well as Gestalt and cognitive-behavioral methods, he began to shape an approach that had at its heart a valuing of inner freedom and personal responsibility. Its humanistic optimism holds the unlimited potential of human functioning and personal growth. He began to focus on how two persons could achieve greater depth in their relationships.

As these theoretical developments unfolded, a life-altering event occurred: we met each other during the first days of our doctoral program. Now our work and relationship began to meld. Not only would we marry within six months of that meeting, but we would also embark on creating our own optimal relationship. We began our practice of couple therapy together, studied other approaches and research in the field, used our relationship as a laboratory for testing our ideas, and applied everything we were learning in our therapeutic work with clients.

As we, along with our clients, experienced the intensity of the closeness we were discovering was possible, we found that the term *voltage* emerged as a fitting description of the energy that every relationship holds. For those who desire a low level of intimacy, with limited or little emotional closeness, the term *low voltage* seemed appropriate. Our clients agreed. For those who desire deep emotional closeness and the intensity of intimacy possible between two people, the term *high voltage* seemed apt. Its valence and hyperbolic nature were captivating. However, as we observed our clients attempting to handle the voltage, and as we ourselves engaged in its creation, we soon realized that skills would be needed. It became apparent that mastering powerful interpersonal skills would be insufficient. To achieve the optimality of high voltage, partners would need to plumb the depths of their own psyches to gain consciousness, insight, and executive mastery of its mysteries. Without such intrapsychic work, the relationship would be highjacked by subconscious processes of which neither partner would be aware.

An interesting dynamic became apparent as we worked with couples. Humans have varying capacity for high-voltage relating. Some people can tolerate high-voltage relating for only minutes as a time. Others can sustain such intensity for the first few weeks or months of a relationship. Very few could not tolerate it at all. This suggested to us that humans seem to naturally dip into this functioning from time to time. Surprisingly, we naturally evidence optimality at some point. However, to sustain optimality for a lifetime occurs rarely. Moreover, a technology for creating and sustaining it has never been formalized.

Creating Optimal Relationships is such formalization. We offer it to equip therapists who are on the front line of helping couples. It is our intention that the values, concepts, and skills of the HVR model guide therapists not only to bring relief to couples in conflict or despair but more profoundly to empower couples for optimal loving for a lifetime.

Creating Optimal Relationships lays out the overview of the voltage approach. The book proceeds by offering a definition of the HVR, along with checklists therapists may use to begin to utilize this model with couple clients. Because the model draws on a theoretical approach that is new to the couple therapy field, Chapter 2 is devoted to orienting the reader to Anthetic Psychology. The remainder of Part 1 explains in detail two major contributions of this approach. First is our discovery of the Inner Critic's sabotaging role in relationship distress, along with innovative clinical strategies to equip couples with skills for becoming free of its influence. Second is the concept of Anthetic Inner Figure work with couples. Part 2 focuses on creating the HVR serves as a handbook for therapists. It offers foundational values couples need, along with the intrapersonal and interpersonal skills used to equip couples to reduce negativity and to achieve optimal relating. Chapter 11 addresses the clinical perspective needed for handling the Voltage Mismatch in couples. Finally, the book concludes with additional skills for maintaining high-voltage relating for a lifetime.

Creating Optimal Relationships is the culmination of a lifetime of work. James began this work in the 1960s in Berkeley, California. He explored it further throughout his forty-year career as a couple therapist. Our exploration continued together in a very personal way throughout our twenty-two-year marriage to each other. A few months prior to suffering a devastating stroke in 2008, James completed the original manuscript from which this one is drawn. Following his death in 2011, I, Kathryn, took up the book once again and have had the joy of completing it for publication. Our work together has been devoted to helping couples bring deep closeness to their relationships. This work is our way to contribute what we discovered to the field of couple therapy and to our fellow therapists.

Part I

A NEW MODEL FOR RELATIONSHIPS

Chapter 1

What is the High-Voltage Relationship?

Expectations pulse through every therapeutic encounter in couple therapy. Perhaps in no other therapeutic endeavor, not individual therapy nor group therapy, does the client enter the process with so much depending on the outcome. Not only does the personal happiness of each partner depend upon the proper functioning of the relationship, but other factors also are contingent on it, including mental health, personal safety, physical health, and even life expectancy (Bloom, Asher, & White, 1978; Burman & Margolin, 1992). Moreover, the couple does not stand isolated in the ramifications of their functioning. Their children also are affected in terms of mental health, developmental progress, social functioning, and even longevity (Gottman, 1999). It therefore is essential that the therapist have a clear sense of what outcome expectancy to hold toward the therapeutic enterprise as well as to offer to the couple.

From the outset, it is essential that one myth in the couple therapy field be dispelled regarding expectations, that is, that high expectations for marriage cause divorce (Lederer & Jackson, 1968). This perspective posited that if couples had lower expectations, they would not become disappointed and so would avoid divorce. However, research has systematically dispelled this myth (Baucom, Epstein, Rankin, & Burnett, 1996) and found instead that the opposite is true. Couples who held higher expectations for their marriages and for romance had the best marriages. The results led to the recommendation that couples should hold uncompromising romantic ideals for marriage (Wile, 1992).

Wile's recommendation naturally suggests the question: is the romantic ideal realistic in terms of actual attainment? According to Acavedo and Aron (2009), the answer is Yes. In analyzing over twenty-five longitudinal and cross-sectional studies of marital satisfaction, researchers found that contrary to conventional professional belief, long-term, intense, engaging, romantic love is a real phenomenon.

Humans are made for romantic love (Aron, Fisher, Mashek, Strong, Haifang, & Brown, 2005). Moreover, countering previous conventional and professional theory, research now shows that the intense euphoria of early-stage romantic love can continue for a lifetime (Aron, et al., 2005). The human brain, in fact, thrives on love across the life span, with longer time in-love subjects exhibiting similar brain function patterns to those in early stage love relationships.

Yet, as central as love is to human experience, only since the 1980s has a field emerged specifically to study relationships, that is, the field of relationship science. From these studies, a body of research is emerging offering findings on closeness and intimacy in personal relationships (see Duck, 1997; Fletcher & Clark, 2000; Kelley, Berscheid, Christensen, Harvey, Huston, Levinger, 1983; and Mashek & Aron, 2004 for compendia of findings). These findings will be drawn upon throughout this book.

Given that the field of relationship science points to what is possible for human relationships; that is, that human physiology can maintain the intensity and gratification of early love, the baton is passed to the field of marital therapy to devise and articulate strategies to support couples in maintaining the optimality of which their brains are capable. Important contributions have been made to apply research findings to marital therapy, among them John Gottman's research on predicting and preventing divorce (Gottman, 1999) and Susan Johnson's *Emotionally Focused Therapy for Couples* (Greenberg & Johnson, 1988; Johnson, 2004), which offers the concept of immediate attention to emotion, along with softening of partners to one another. Despite these clinical advances, optimality as a goal has not been the focus of marital therapy.

Perhaps professionals have doubted the ability of marriage to contain the bliss Acavedo and Aron described because the field of marriage and family therapy has lacked an adequate model for helping couples to achieve it. This book offers a new model called the High-Voltage Relationship (HVR). Its goal is to equip therapists with both an ideal to guide their practice and a skills-based approach enabling couples to achieve and sustain the optimality; even bliss previously thought impossible.

INTEGRATION OF TWO KINDS OF SKILL: OPTIMAL RELATING AND PSYCHOLOGICAL GROWTH

The high-voltage model is based on the following principle: What is needed for a satisfying relationship is an integrated combination of two kinds of skill.

First, the couple needs skills for optimal relating and, second, the couple requires skills for each partner's psychological growth. Such psychological growth skills are necessary to create the right infrastructure to support the optimal relating skills. In over forty years of clinical research with hundreds of interpersonal groups and over a thousand couples, the authors found that when couples learned and used these two kinds of skill, not only did longevity of their relationship result, but also a level of couple functioning that surpassed ordinary marital satisfaction. These skills equipped the couple to achieve what could be called *optimal relating*. The term *optimal* seems fitting because it describes the factors that have emerged in couple research as essential in either preventing divorce or increasing happiness. These factors include feelings of closeness and "feeling loved" (Gigy and Kelly, 1992), resolution of the symbolic meaning in partner conflict (Gottman, 1999), and self-expansion through partner interdependence (Rusbult, Kumashiro, Stocker, Kirchner, Finkel and Coolsen, 2005). In other words, utilizing the skills enabled partners not only to resolve conflict, but also to feel loved and emotionally close to their partners, and even to feel they were attaining their ideal selves.

Why "High-Voltage"?

While the term *high voltage* can hold associations for some as being overly intense and somehow dangerous, the authors chose the term to assist clients in visualizing the soulful potential awaiting them in their relationships. In contrast to current relationship models which offer conflict resolution, dysfunction reduction, divorce prevention, or mere fondness as the goal (Gottman, 1999; Johnson, 2004; Sweeney, Ziskind, & Schwartz, 2013), the high-voltage model offers extraordinary depth, emotional closeness, and intensity.

High Voltage as a Goal

What makes the HVR so desirable to many people can be seen in one nearly infallible test: The high-voltage person is one who hungers for depth and emotional closeness in conversations with others. While high-voltage persons can engage in routine small talk, especially as a friendly beginning, soon they want something more. In short, the high-voltage person longs for a depth connection, in which he or she can talk with his or her partner about anything, not holding back any relevant thoughts, feelings, or requests. Such depth requires skills for managing feelings that emerge when conversations involve revelation of inner material in each partner. HVR skills in clinical practice have empowered couples to create a deep emotional bond that becomes the context for the emergence of powerful love and blissful connection. The HVR is also characterized by such values as responsibility, mutuality, compassion, and affectionate love and caring.

The Low-Voltage Relationship

While the benefits of the HVR seem so desirable that one might assume that most couples would want more closeness, clinical experience revealed that this was not a universal desire. Some couples wanted a more surface relationship and were content with greater distance between them. Low-voltage partners valued more formality, conventionality, and rigidity of relating. They preferred to live more as roommates rather than as the soul mates to which HVR couples aspired. These couples fit a Low-Voltage Relationship (LVR) model marked by much less emotional intensity. With such couples, minimal skills could be taught to reduce any conflict or difficulty that brought them to therapy. As clinical research progressed, the voltage concept proved useful in giving couples specific terms for articulating the kind of relationship they wanted.

DISTINGUISHING HIGH-VOLTAGE AND LOW-VOLTAGE RELATING

Perhaps the most unusual distinction between HVRs and LVRs is that high-voltage partners live what can be termed a psychologically principled life; that is, a life grounded on principles that are based on a psychological infrastructure. High-voltage partners choose to address their problems through psychological work on themselves and the employment of interpersonal skills for directly addressing conflict. While such strategies involving directly addressing partner feelings and psychodynamic motivations may lead to some initial discomfort, these partners value the satisfying resolutions that result. Couples report greater happiness that they describe as going far beyond ordinary pleasantness.

In contrast, low-voltage partners in choosing surface relating, often evade problems. While they may live a principled life, the principles are not psychologically based. Because of this, low-voltage partners often pursue their relationships by following a rigid set of meticulously ordered rules. This pursuit often results in simmering resentments with which the couple never deals. The result can be seen on a continuum of relationship functioning from distant cordiality to freely expressed negativity to intense relational combat to leaving.

This does not mean that low-voltage partners cannot achieve a modicum of happiness and stability. They may do so through bypassing couple problems and avoiding hot topics. Strategies for achieving such stability include humorizing through saying funny things and by limiting their conversation to surface topics. The partners may in fact live as fun-loving roommates.

Creating the High-Voltage Relationship

For partners who desire an HVR, the therapist can guide them to consciously design their relationship according to three foundational steps. These three foundations prepare the couple to view their relationship as a personal development school for their own psychological growth. Specifically, partners must choose to foster a safe haven where they can combine deep and loving closeness with the growth methods that are needed to support that closeness. A safe haven has been described in the literature (Johnson, 2004) as a relationship in which partners can let down their everyday defenses in order to reveal vulnerable feelings. HVR skills have been developed so that couples may possess doable skills for relating to each other in order to maintain a climate of non-judgmental acceptance and empathy. This book develops in detail the three foundations for learning to create an HVR:

- Foundation 1: These are the basic guidelines, that is, values, concepts, and principles necessary for understanding the intrapersonal and interpersonal skills that come later.
- Foundation 2: These are the intrapersonal skills the therapist teaches partners so they may do psychological work on themselves.
- Foundation 3: These are the interpersonal skills, specifically step-by-step instructions for high-voltage communicating.

Mastery of Foundations 1, 2, and 3 is sequential. If a couple finds it difficult to employ the Foundation 3 interpersonal communication skills, the therapist can infer that they have not learned the Foundation 2 intrapersonal skills. If the partners have difficulty doing the intrapersonal skills for their own psychological work, the therapist can surmise that they have not learned the Foundation 1 basic guidelines.

In other words, this book offers an integrated program. If the couple desires an LVR, it is possible for the therapist to teach those interpersonal communication skills needed for smoother conventional surface relating. However, if the couple would like an HVR, the therapist will need to teach the couple all three foundation elements.

Once the therapist has helped the couple learn the elements of Foundations 1, 2, and 3, couple problems become an opportunity for partners' personal growth and the couple's optimal relating. Moreover, for those partners in a romantic relationship, the HVR then becomes a haven for romantic love, which according to American Psychological Association research is associated with greater relationship satisfaction (Acevedo & Aron, 2009).

Important Distinctions: What the High-Voltage Relationship is *Not*

In order to refine the definition of the HVR, clarification of the term is essential. Following is a list of items to distinguish the HVR from any relationship elements that it is *not*:

1. *It is not simply dramatic feelings and energetic activities.* Instead, the HVR is at its heart about depth and emotional closeness, which may not be dramatic at all. In addition, there may be no energetic activities involved in it.
2. *It is not merely sexuality.* There is a temptation to see the HVR in terms of good sex. However, there may be no sexual intimacy at all between the partners. For example, HVRs can occur not only between spouses but also between friends, relatives, and between parents and their adult children.
3. *It is not confined to the expression of a great deal of love between partners.* Individuals who have a strong desire to be loved may be tempted to think of the HVR simply as a means for obtaining supplies of that love. Although high-voltage partners may give and receive intense love, the HVR is also about caring and closeness, which, as the authors will explain, are not identical with love.
4. *It is not simply talking a lot.* Although high-voltage partners do spend a lot of time talking to each other, the HVR is not just about talking a lot. The important element that defines high voltage is not the amount of time spent talking. It is instead whether what is said is superficial or comes from the heart. It is the depth at which the talking takes place. To achieve this depth, the couple's communication is guided by the value of honesty rather than looking good to each other. An example of depth communication is, "You're right. When I said that, I was being defensive."
5. *It is not merely a passionate desire to be together.* High-voltage people, whether in a relationship with a friend, or a relative (parent, child, or other), or a romantic partner often like to spend a lot of time together, but time together does not in itself make the relationship high voltage. In fact, partners can have an HVR without much proximity at all.

Distilling the Essential Elements of the High-Voltage Relationship

While it will be the work of the entire book to lay out the elements of the HVR, what can be offered here is the one essential element that is the core feature of the HVR, that is, *emotional closeness*. Later will follow a special definition of closeness, along with the elements it comprises. At this point, it is important to state that emotional closeness occurs when partners share thoughts and feelings openly and honesty, connect directly to what the other has said, and provide involved responses from a soft-hearted attitude.

HIGH-VOLTAGE AND LOW-VOLTAGE MARRIAGES

An important benefit of the voltage concept in defining relationships is its usefulness in assessing partner compatibility. When two individuals both desire a great deal of emotional closeness, they are said to want an HVR. In contrast, when both partners desire much less closeness and want a surface relationship, they can be said to have a low-voltage marriage.

The low-voltage marriage is marked by parallel relating. Partners engage in side-by-side activities and conversations about activities or other people but do not converse about their own relationship. The LVR can be satisfying and stable, provided partners maintain sufficient distance from each other. The relationship can be a reasonably comfortable one, despite the loneliness that is associated with it.

The high-voltage marriage is distinguished by the depth of emotional content involved in partner conversation. Most important, the couple engages in analysis of their relationship, discussing feelings for each other as well as perspective on the state of their relationship.

The Voltage Mismatch

When partners are matched in terms of voltage desires, their relationships usually contain more satisfaction. Frequently however partners present as having disparate voltage desires. One partner wants high-voltage relating and the other desires low voltage. These couples are said to have a voltage mismatch. In the authors' clinical experience such couples typically seek counseling for puzzling conflict. In the literature on couples counseling, these partners are labeled as exhibiting the pursuer/distance pattern, also called demand/withdraw pattern (Christenson, 1987, 1988; Christenson & Heavey, 1990). When the clinician explains the concepts of high and low voltage, the couple is often relieved to understand the source of their conflict.

A High-Voltage and Low-Voltage Marriage

Consider the case of Ellen and Dan, married two years, with no children. Ellen worked as an elementary school teacher. She functioned in relationship as a high-voltage partner. She craved connection at deep levels. Dan was a lawyer, who was the head of his own firm. When the voltage concept was introduced by the therapist, he identified himself as high voltage because he was aggressive in the courtroom. He was surprised to discover that he functioned as a low-voltage partner in intimate relationships. He avoided emotional closeness.

Ellen and Dan sought therapy because of ongoing conflict about Dan's unwillingness to open up. In the beginning months of their marriage, they both experienced a great deal of love and closeness. However, the love and closeness soon diminished significantly. As Dan built his law practice, he spent more and more time at work. Ellen reported feeling lonely. After months of misery, Ellen demanded that Dan join her in couple counseling. Dan was reluctant but decided to attend after Ellen told him she was considering divorce.

In their initial session, Ellen spoke first. "I think we have communication problems," she said. "I want something more out of my marriage, but I don't know whether I have the right to ask for it, and I'm not even sure what it is. When we were dating, Dan was very attentive. He brought me flowers. He told me he loved me. He showered me with affection. He even sent me little love notes. We talked and talked for hours about everything under the sun. Then the moment we said 'I do,' everything changed. He started to stay late at his office. He spent a lot of time working on his computer. He went out with his friends, drinking, and I wasn't invited. I felt miserable. Lonely."

"I agree; it's a communication problem," Dan said. "I don't know what she's complaining about. I make over $500,000 a year from my law practice. We have two expensive cars. We live in a luxury house. She has everything she wants. I'm so busy working with people all day, I need some time by myself when I get home. What did that guy write? I need to go into my cave. I get enough conflict in my work. All I want is to be left alone. She's immature. She has unrealistic expectations about marriage. It's not all that fireworks stuff that it started out with. She's always unhappy with me. I want to be accepted for who I am, not badgered into being someone I'm not."

In conceptualizing the distress Ellen and Dan presented, common elements of the HV-LV relationship were evident:

1. The relationship began with high intensity during the courting stage. Both partners wanted that intensity and liked it.
2. The voltage began to decline right after the wedding. Ellen was unhappy with the decline; Dan attempted to legitimize it by saying it was just human nature. Dan tried to persuade Ellen that the decline was not a

problem. This led Ellen to become self-doubting, to question her desire for more emotional closeness. She did not know with any certainty what was normal. She wondered if Dan were right in saying that her expectations were too high for continued intensity in marriage.

3. The couple thought their problem was one of communication, not values. If only they could learn the right communication skills, they believed, they could improve their marriage.
4. Ellen wanted more depth and intensity. The more she tried to get it, however, the more Dan tried to persuade her that it was unreasonable. That is, he invoked the principle of reasonableness instead of stating a preference. He implied there was something wrong in principle with wanting so much intensity. He then added a judgmental assessment that Ellen was immature. He did not say, "I prefer less intensity; you prefer more, but there's nothing wrong with either of us."
5. Dan wanted to be left alone. The more he tried to get it, the more Ellen tried to persuade him that it was an unreasonable request. She invoked the principle of reasonableness also, instead of simply stating a preference. Her position was, "Marriage should be a deep and intense relationship." She could not say, "I prefer more intensity; you prefer less, but there's nothing wrong with either of us."
6. Dan invoked a relationship writer to support his case. As a result of reading this author, Dan felt justified in "going into his cave." Ellen did not have an expert to invoke to support her desire for more emotional closeness.
7. Dan, the low-voltage partner, could not see what Ellen was unhappy about. He thought the marriage was going along just fine. He thought the problem could be solved if Ellen would stop nagging him.
8. Dan simply wanted to be accepted the way he was. He could not understand why he did not get that acceptance. He did not realize that he in turn could not accept Ellen's desire for more intimacy.
9. Dan did not want to begin counseling. "There's nothing really wrong with our relationship," he thought. "Sooner or later she'll settle down just like my mom did and be satisfied with the marriage." He came to counseling to please her. He did not think he needed to do any changing.
10. In counseling, as in the marriage, Dan was reluctant to talk about his feelings. He did not think talking about feelings could help. Nor did he think counseling could help.
11. Not only did Dan dislike intense intimacy, he felt judgmental toward what he labeled "touchy-feely" interactions.
12. Dan's work was conflict-ridden, challenging, and demanding. He did not want to have to deal with any conflict at home in addition to his other problems.

13. Ellen felt defective. Her self-doubt prevented her from saying with strong conviction what she really wanted. She could not even admit it to herself. She did know that she did not want things to go on the way they were. She needed help formulating her wishes.
14. Dan's vision of marriage was one in which his chief role was to provide a good living from his work.
15. Dan had no idea what Ellen was complaining about. He lacked concepts for understanding her perspective.

    Ellen said, "Let's get couple counseling."

    Dan replied, "No. We don't need to run to a counselor every time we have a problem. We can solve our problems ourselves. Let's just put this behind us, start over, and try harder to get along by not upsetting each other."

In order to help Ellen and Dan understand the dynamic that was functioning in their relationship, the therapists offered them six checklists for each to answer, the *Checklist for High-Voltage Relating, Checklist of Low-Voltage Principles, Checklist of Low-Voltage Communication, Statements that Indicate a Preference for Low-Voltage Relationships, Low-Voltage Behavior During an Argument,* and *Checklist for Interest/Involvement* (see all below). Ellen's answers on the *High-Voltage Relating* checklist were all True; Dan answered True to only Items #2 and #6. On the *Checklist of Low-Voltage Principles,* both of their answers were 90 percent indicative that their marriage was functioning as a low voltage one. Their answers on the *Checklist for Low-Voltage Communication* indicated they primarily communicated in a low-voltage style. Dan's answers on *Statements that Indicate a Preference for Low-Voltage Relationships, Low Voltage Behavior During an Argument,* and *Checklist for Interest/Involvement* were consistently indicative of Low-voltage relating, while Ellen's indicated high voltage. As partners, their profile pointed to a voltage discrepancy, the classic voltage mismatch.

During the discussion of their answers with the therapists, Ellen said, "This explains my frustration. I like high-voltage relating and Dan likes low-voltage." Dan said, "Thinking of us as wanting two different kinds of relationship sure puts a new spin on our problems." Ellen added, "Yes, and now I see that we started out relating in a high-voltage way. That suited me just right. But now we've fallen into low-voltage relating, and that's why I'm so unhappy." Dan agreed, "I liked when we were close before, but I thought from watching my Mom and Dad and others that you just couldn't keep that closeness up. Is it really possible to do that?"

The therapists assured Dan and Ellen that the level of voltage they desired was now their choice to make. Therapy would assist them with the skills for the level of voltage they chose.

CHECKLIST FOR HIGH-VOLTAGE RELATING

This test is for you to assess your desire for an HVR with a spouse, lover, relative, or friend. Note again that the word "partner" refers to all four categories.

Directions: Please circle "**T**" if you think the statement generally applies to you or "**F**" if you think it does not.

1. I like to talk to my partner about our relationship. **T F**
2. I like to make up quickly after an argument. **T F**
3. I like to read self-help books on relationships. **T F**
4. I like to tell my partner "I love you" or (a friend) "I like you." **T F**
5. When we have a problem, I want to discuss it as soon as possible. **T F**
6. I would be willing to get into counseling with my partner. **T F**
7. I like to talk about my feelings. **T F**
8. I'd like to listen to my partner talk about his or her feelings. **T F**
9. I don't like a lot of surface talk. **T F**
10. With my partner, I'm open with what I'm thinking and feeling. **T F**
11. With my partner, I never say "That's none of your business" or "I don't want to talk about it." **T F**
12. With my partner, I never say "I don't have to tell her I love her. She knows it already." **T F**
13. I like to tell my partner about his or her good qualities. **T F**
14. I like to analyze our conversations and arguments. **T F**

Scoring: If you circled every **T** you prefer high-voltage relating. If you circled only a few **T**'s, or none at all, you more than likely prefer low-voltage relating.

CHECKLIST OF LOW-VOLTAGE PRINCIPLES

Directions: Circle the items as True or False, corresponding to principles that either you or your partner are applying to your relationship.

1. Don't try to change your partner; just work on changing yourself. **T F**
2. If you want too much closeness, your partner will feel smothered; so it is better to back off. **T F**
3. You can't keep the romance (or intensity) you had when you first met. It naturally declines. **T F**
4. Anger is nothing to work on. It is just an emotion that comes and goes as it will. **T F**

5. One partner needs to go into his cave from time to time. The other partner should cultivate other hobbies and interests. **T F**
6. If your partner is angry or judgmental toward you, just overlook it. **T F**
7. Don't give your partner feedback or "take your partner's inventory." **T F**
8. Partners must grow up and forget about having a deeply satisfying relationship or a thrilling romantic marriage. Those relationships are found only in fairytales. **T F**
9. A good way to solve a conflict is just not to talk about it; it will usually then solve itself. **T F**
10. Being honest with your partner is usually not a good idea; it might upset him or her. **T F**
11. Don't tell your partner what you want if it will hurt his or her feelings. **T F**
12. Don't ask your partner too many personal questions. **T F**
13. Don't analyze your arguments; just let them be what they are. **T F**
14. Going to couple counseling means you are mentally disturbed or abnormal. **T F**
15. You ought to be able to handle things on your own. **T F**

Scoring: The principles listed above are those that produce low-voltage relating. The more items you circle as True, the more likely you prefer LVRs.

CHECKLIST OF LOW-VOLTAGE COMMUNICATION

High-voltage couples engage in honest, direct, open communication. This is the core of the HVR. Low-voltage couples have decided not to be always open and honest. They have not yet learned the skills to handle the intensity that comes from honesty, directness, and openness.

Directions: Circle the items below as True or False that apply to your communication style:

1. There are some things I need to talk about but that I'm too embarrassed to discuss with my partner. **T F**
2. I don't share all my important thoughts and feelings with my partner because if I did, he or she would get upset. **T F**
3. Usually, if I feel hurt in response to something my partner said or did, I don't tell my partner. **T F**
4. There are some things I'm afraid to ask my partner for. **T F**
5. Sometimes I'm afraid to tell my partner when I'm angry. **T F**
6. If my partner wants to do something, and I don't, sometimes I'm afraid to say so. **T F**

7. There are some things I'm afraid to say because I might get a judgmental reply or might be verbally punished by my partner. **T F**
8. There are some topics I can't bring up, because my partner wouldn't like it. **T F**
9. Sometimes I don't give my opinion, because my partner wouldn't consider it rationally and objectively but would just reject it. **T F**

Scoring: The more items you've circled as "**T**," the more likely it is that your communication style is low voltage.

STATEMENTS THAT INDICATE A PREFERENCE FOR LOW-VOLTAGE RELATIONSHIPS

One indicator of a preference for low-voltage relating is what a partner believes about relationships in general and their own in particular.

Directions: Check the items with which you agree:

1. ___I don't see much point in talking about feelings.
2. ___I don't like to read books about the psychology of relationships.
3. ___I wish people would stop giving me all that psychological garbage.
4. ___I don't want to go to couple counseling.
5. ___I told my spouse I loved him or her when we got married, so I wish he or she would stop asking me all the time.
6. ___Our relationship is what it is. I don't want to talk about it.
7. ___I don't like to analyze things to death. I prefer to go with the flow.
8. ___I am who I am. I'm not going to change.
9. ___I don't like touchy feely stuff.
10. ___My partner wants too much from me.
11. ___I think my partner is an intensity junkie.

Scoring: The more items you checked, the more likely it is that you prefer LVRs.

Low-Voltage Behavior during an Argument

How a partner handles an argument can indicate whether he or she prefers low voltage. You can use this checklist of argument behaviors to decide if you function from a low-voltage position.

Directions: Check the following items you have said during an argument (or at any time):

1. ____ You're too sensitive.
2. ____ I need my space. You're too intrusive.
3. ____ That's my business, not yours; don't be so nosy.
4. ____ You're too emotional.
5. ____ You take things too seriously.
6. ____ You're just too thin-skinned. Toughen up.
7. ____ Your expectations for marriage are too high.
8. ____ Let's just put this behind us and start over.
9. ____ Don't be so serious. Let's keep it light.
10. ____ Stop analyzing things to death.
11. ____ I don't want to work at reducing my anger; that's just me.
12. ____ When my partner asks me to work on my anger, I get even more angry.

Scoring: The more check marks you have made, the more likely you function from a low-voltage position.

Checklist for Interest/Involvement

One of the best indicators of high-voltage relating is how much interest and involvement partners have with each other.

Directions: Check the items that are true:

1. ____ My partner frequently asks me questions about my likes and dislikes.
2. ____ My partner knows the kind of work I like to do.
3. ____ My partner knows about the traumatic events of my life.
4. ____ My partner knows about the happiest times of my life.
5. ____ My partner knows about the major decisions, turning points, and defining moments in my life.
6. ____ My partner knows which talents and accomplishments I am most happy to have.
7. ____ My partner knows the kinds of music I like.
8. ____ My partner knows the kinds of books I like to read.
9. ____ My partner knows what I like to watch on TV.
10. ____ My partner knows what I like to listen to on the radio.
11. ____ My partner knows about my vocational or career goals.
12. ____ My partner knows my favorite foods and restaurants.
13. ____ My partner knows my religious beliefs.
14. ____ When my partner gives me gifts, he or she selects them thoughtfully to make sure they're what I would really like.

15. ____ My partner knows about my hobbies and interests.
16. ____ My partner knows my entertainment likes and dislikes.
17. ____ My partner knows the places I like to go on vacation.
18. ____ My partner knows my recreational likes and dislikes.
19. ____ My partner knows about my fears.
20. ____ My partner knows about my physical and medical problems.
21. ____ My partner can easily say what he or she likes about me.

And finally, for a romantic relationship:

22. ____ My partner knows what I like (and don't like) sexually.
23. ____ My partner knows what I like when it comes to demonstrations of affection.

Scoring: Low-voltage partners do not know much about their partners, whereas the communication intensity of the HVR lends itself to partners learning a great deal about each other. The fewer check marks made in the above checklist, the more likely that the partners are engaging in an LVR. The more check marks, the more likely the partners have an HVR.

The six checklists above can be used by the clinician early in the therapeutic process. As the therapist and couple discuss the results of each checklist, partners are able to see the level of voltage from which they have been functioning. In addition, the results are useful in kindling partners' discussion of their satisfaction or dissatisfaction with the level of voltage they have in their relationship. It may also be quite helpful at that point, for the clinician to offer both advantages and disadvantages that correlate with each level of voltage.

LOW-VOLTAGE RELATIONSHIP

Advantages of the Low-Voltage Relationship

One might think that all the relationship advantages lie with the HVR. Not so. There are some interesting advantages in having a LVR, provided both partners want it:

1. Since partners in the LVR do not talk much, and do not communicate in depth at all, there may be little or no apparent conflict, as long as both partners maintain a great deal of distance between each other, are satisfied with that distance, and maintain a climate of politeness.
2. Because there is little depth communication, it is easy for partners to keep secrets from one another. In the LVR it is not unusual for partners to be

unaware when one of them has seen a counselor or an attorney or even is having an affair.
3. The LVR is ideal for partners who fall into the self-sufficient type (to be explained in detail in Chapter 3). These are partners who prefer to do things alone much of the time.
4. Partners often feel less anxiety, in that they do not take risks of self-disclosure.
5. Partners have a great deal of freedom to do whatever each wants, without being concerned about what the other partner wants. Therefore, the challenge of negotiating differences is minimized.

Low-Voltage Skills

Low-voltage partners who seek counseling for relief from distress occurring in the relationship have a more limited goal than high-voltage clients; therefore, the therapist's interventions are typically more limited. Among the interpersonal skills found helpful for low-voltage couples are *Anthetic Requesting, Anthetic Listening,* and *Empathizing* (explained in Chapters 9 and 10). Intrapersonal skills the authors have found valuable for LVR functioning include *Slowing Down, Relaxing,* and *Self-Soothing* (Chapter 6). These skills when taught alone have been useful in resolving conflict while maintaining the distance that low-voltage couples prefer.

Disadvantages of the Low-Voltage Relationship

Many couples have achieved successful LVR. However, there are several disadvantages inherent in the LVR.

1. The LVR can be lonely. The less Self-Sufficient Low-Voltage partner may find this loneliness painful.
2. There may be a great deal of misunderstandings. Because the partners do not like to talk much, they may misinterpret each other's statements, which may lead to a great deal of arguments.
3. As long as the couple experiences no crises, the relationship may go along smoothly. However, relationships are known for their crises. Clinical practice has revealed twenty-one of the most common ones: having a baby; having problems with in-laws; loss of a job by one partner; serious illness or disability of a partner or a child; death of a child; death of a parent; sexual or emotional infidelity; children growing up and leaving home; arrest for and conviction of a crime; loss of interest in sex; one partner wanting to change his or her religion; disagreements about where to live; severe emotional withdrawal of a partner; mental illness; substance abuse; change

in a partner's sexual orientation or gender identity; a problem with a child; a relative moving into the home; bitter disagreements about how to raise children; unemployment; loss of money in investments; and bankruptcy. Low-voltage partners have a great deal of difficulty handling these crises.

4. Moreover, it is difficult for partners in LVR to resolve even minor problems. Because partners operate from the principle embodied in the statement, "Let's just put our problems behind us and try harder not to upset each other," the content and any underlying dynamics within the problem are not addressed.
5. Communication becomes difficult. Without high-voltage communication skills, the couple finds their problems escalating, at times to the point of considering ending the relationship.
6. LVRs often contain a power differential. In the relationship, differences of opinion are often handled by one partner deciding and the other going along with the decision, even if that decision is not liked.
7. Partners are less likely to be getting what they want, whether less significant items such as birthday and Christmas gifts or emotionally vital support such as being present during childbirth or a parent's dying.
8. If the relationship is LV-LV, there is no voltage disparity. The relationship may be able to coast for years without any serious problems. However, serious problems can upset the equilibrium the couple has achieved. In addition, a surprising disequilibrium can occur when one partner experiences a whiff of an HVR and decides to leave the other partner for a deeper relationship.

Additional Problems with the Low-Voltage Relationship

Because the LVR style involves living like roommates, one might think the relationship can turn out to be satisfying, similar to good relationships between college roommates. Such relationships in college may have involved fondness between the roommates but more often than not no love for each other. Neither expected much closeness and did not complain if they did not receive it. Each had their own friends and activities. Therefore, applying the roommate model might lead to the conclusion that the LVR could be manageable though somewhat distant. However, low-voltage couples have provided numerous examples of difficulties that occur within the LVR:

- One person says something, and the other ignores it.
- An important decision must be made, and one partner does not want to talk about it.
- One partner makes a major decision without first consulting with the other partner.

- One person gets angry and has no skills to process it. The other partner feels deeply hurt, and the pain remains unresolved. Such pain may turn into a permanent grudge, coloring everything that is said from that time on.
- One partner will not talk. The other partner tries to open him or her up by being judgmental. The quiet partner withdraws even more. The tension becomes electric. That night they each sleep on their own side of the bed or one person sleeps on the couch.
- One partner does not say what he or she wants. Over time, this partner's needs remain unmet. Finally, the partner leaves instead of saying what he or she wants. In one case, the partner left a note propped against the sugar bowl: "I'm getting a divorce. Don't try to find me."
- Because there is no commitment to honesty, one partner lies and gets caught, then shrugs it off, saying, "It was just a little thing, and I didn't want to upset you."
- Neither partner has the skills needed for resolving conflicts, and each winds up with painful feelings. The result is that the conflict never gets resolved.
- Anxiety and depression often accompany the pain of the LVR. Because the couple does not see that the source of the depression is the relationship, it is treated by medication. The interpersonal conflict remains unresolved.
- When low-voltage partners reach a certain level of unhappiness, they may reject the option of marriage counseling and decide to divorce, with serious consequences for the children.

HIGH-VOLTAGE RELATIONSHIP

Advantages of the High-Voltage Relationship

Couple clients who have chosen to work toward an HVR report that while it may not be easy to achieve, the HVR is enormously satisfying. Roberta, an oncologist, said, "I didn't know there was such a thing as an HVR, but now that I know, I can see why my ex-husband and I had so many arguments. I wanted closeness, he didn't. Now, I wouldn't even consider low-voltage relating. High-voltage is what I wanted all along, but I didn't know it. My relationship with my ex was like black and white movies. With my new husband, it's like Technicolor."

Following are additional advantages of the HVR the authors have observed:

1. Because it liberates emotional energies, HVR couples report feeling joyous and even ecstatic.
2. Because it is playful and passionate, the HVR keeps love and romance alive.

3. The HVR is exciting. It engenders creativity. Couples report being surprised by the pleasure they create together.
4. Because HVR skills are specifically aimed at helping couples resolve conflict, couples report that crises that often occur in relationships can more easily be overcome.
5. Because the HVR produces emotional highs, it reduces the couple's need for chemical highs through drugs or alcohol. The authors have demonstrated its effectiveness in chemical dependency relapse prevention (Elliott, 2006).
6. The HVR has the potential to stimulate partners' psychological growth, as every couple problem is seen as a lesson to be learned.
7. Because of the honesty, depth communication, and emotional closeness entailed in the HVR, the risk of infidelity is reduced.

Disadvantages of the High-Voltage Relationship

The HVR does not happen automatically. Nor does it happen simply by loving the other person enough. Instead it requires that partners engage in psychological work on themselves.

1. The psychological work partners do may trigger feelings of anxiety. The anxiety results from the disconfirmation of each person's self-image as each faces elements within themselves or how they relate.
2. In working on their own psychodynamic issues, partners experience regression in the service of growth; what Kris (1952) called "regression in the service of the ego." Early in the process, each partner's level of executive self-functioning (akin to ego strength) will be called on and challenged. For some with little executive functioning, decompensation may occur, with resulting feelings of anxiety or depression. (The model addresses this event first by equipping partners with skills for challenging Inner Critic messages which fuel the decompensation. The therapist assists the partner to utilize Inner Critic challenging skills for any event of decompensation. These skills are covered in Chapter 3.)
3. Because the HVR is a skills-based approach, it requires partners to spend a considerable amount of time learning the basic guidelines and skills of high-voltage relating contained throughout this book.
4. The HVR requires a great deal of attention to the relationship. Issues and problems are addressed directly using the skills, which may require taking one or two hours of time.
5. Learning the new skills may be difficult for one or both partners, not because the concepts are intellectually rigorous, but because partners may have defense mechanisms triggered as they confront inner material.

Cultural Implications of the High-Voltage Relationship Model

Both neurophysiological research and ethnographic studies indicate that romantic love is a cross-cultural and nearly universal phenomenon. In a survey of 166 contemporary societies, Jankowiak and Fischer (1992) found that romantic love occurred in 147 of them, with the remaining 19 examples appearing to be the result of ethnographic oversight. The intensity of romantic love has been found to involve emotional responses including euphoria, intense focused attention on a chosen individual, obsessive thinking about him or her, cravings for emotional union with the beloved, and increased energy (Fisher, 1998; Gonzaga, Londahl, & Smith, 2001; Harris & Christenfeld, 1996; Hatfield & Sprecher, 1986; Shaver, Schwartz, Kirson, & O'Connor, 1987).

The universality of this human experience appears to have its source in the neurophysiology of the brain of all humans, primarily in basic reward functions and dopamine activation systems (Fisher, 1998; Aron et al., 2004). The research on romantic love has implications regarding the capacity of all humans for HVR, in that the elements of romantic love correlate with the elements of cathexis, closeness, merging, and expansiveness that characterize high voltage.

Because the study of cultural differences regarding closeness is still relatively recent, cultural perspectives are still evolving. However, certain differences have been suggested. For example, while North American cultures emphasize mutual intimate self-disclosure in the definition of closeness, this element is not a powerful determinant of satisfaction in many West African worlds. In such cultures, responsiveness in relationship obligations seems to serve as the basis for intimacy (Laurenceau, Rivera, Schaffer, & Pietromonaco, 2004; Adams, Anderson, & Adonu, 2004).

Regarding implications for the LGBT community, clinical experience indicates that voltage is not related to gender, sexual orientation, or gender identity. Rather, voltage desires are the choice of each individual and each couple.

For those individuals who choose a perspective on closeness consistent with the North American one, culture plays an important role. Cultural legacies can influence partners to hold beliefs about close relationships that may hinder closeness (Schwartz, 1995). Examples include materialism, self-reliance, patriarchy, and racism.

Summary of the High-Voltage Relationship

To summarize, the HVR is based on partners' commitment to using psychotherapeutic growth methods in their everyday conversations. These methods are not meant to imply that partners have mental health problems. The approach is based on the clinical discovery that learning and using high-voltage skills results in emotional closeness between partners. Partners who desire closeness find this model produces a more satisfying life.

In essence the approach holds that a relationship offers the opportunity to become a school for partners' growth by working on their problems. The process of awakening and growth is a lifelong task. In the authors' couple therapy experience of almost half a century, couples who have chosen the high-voltage path have found that the skills soon become second nature and are delightfully enjoyable, resulting in a deeply satisfying relationship.

Chapter 2

A New Psychology as the Foundation for the High-Voltage Relationship

The concept of the HVR has evoked a powerful response in group members as well as in individuals and couples in therapy. More often than not, individuals and couples are attracted to the concept, stating a desire for high-voltage relating. Despite its attractiveness, however, skills alone have proved insufficient as a foundation for functioning at such optimal levels. As initial research in Anthetic T-Groups unfolded (Elliott & Elliott, 2013), it became apparent that group members, as well as individuals and couples, aspiring to relating in a high-voltage way would need a psychological infrastructure to support the new skills that would enable them to engage in high-voltage relating.

After surveying a vast array of schools of conventional (and unconventional) psychology and psychotherapy, it became apparent that none was appropriate for the purpose of laying such a foundation. Accordingly, it became necessary to create a new infrastructure; one based on research the authors conducted with groups. This infrastructure was carefully crafted to serve as the foundational discipline for learning and practicing the high-voltage skills. What emerged was a new growth-oriented psychology with an emphasis on inner freedom. The primacy of inner freedom represented a unique approach not previously seen in the field. The new psychology had as its goal to equip group members to achieve the integration of two disciplines: optimal *interpersonal relating* and *psychological growth*. This integration could be achieved by applying psychotherapeutic principles to everyday relationships.

The new approach was named Anthetic Psychology. The term *Anthetic* was derived from the Greek *anthein,* referring to the growth and blossoming of a flower. Anthetic Psychology holds that once internal obstacles are cleared away and dysfunctional learnings are corrected, the individual is free to grow, unfold, and blossom in his or her own way.

Anthetics then became the fountainhead discipline. It comprises a number of areas of derivative study, including Anthetic Philosophy, Anthetic Therapy, and Anthetic Relationship Therapy. Anthetic Philosophy is a field of study that views philosophizing as a psychological process requiring freedom from psychological reactivity to prevent contamination of the philosophizing process (Elliott & Elliott, 1997). At the same time, Anthetic Philosophy serves as a conceptual architectonics, a foundation for Anthetic Psychology, addressing questions of ontology, axiology, ethics, and epistemology. Anthetic Psychology deals with the study of the human psyche: thoughts, feelings, attitudes, and behavior. Anthetic Therapy concerns itself with applying principles of Anthetic Psychology to human life and the solutions of human problems. Anthetic Relationship Therapy includes the application of Anthetic Therapeutic principles to relationships of all kinds, including intimate partners.

Anthetic Philosophy

Ontologically, Anthetic Philosophy postulates that each individual has at core an essential self called the Transcendental Self or T-self (Elliott & Elliott, 2000). The T-self is who the person is at the core level of being. It is basically an observer. All other elements of the personality are added on to the T-self. This self is similar to Husserl's (1960) transcendental ego or Kant's (1900) transcendental unity of apperception.

Implied from this conceptualization is that partners in relationships bring the essential T-self to the relationship. However, other elements often are salient as features of the personality that have been accrued during development inform or even drive how the partners relate to each other. These elements include inner figures (to be covered further in Chapter 4), beliefs, and other cognitive structures such as judgmentalism (to be discussed in Chapter 9).

Anthetic Psychology

The principles of Anthetic Psychology were influenced by a number of pioneers in the field of psychology, although in every case Elliott radically revised their ideas, omitted much, and added many new concepts and methods (Elliott & Elliott, 2000). Anthetic Psychology differs in important ways from other schools of psychology both in theories of psychopathology and methods of treatment.

The foundational concept used in Anthetic Psychology is the Inner Critic, which is roughly synonymous with the Freudian superego (Freud, 1923/1949a). However, there are important differences. Freud (1914/1949b) saw the superego as composed of two parts: the ego ideal, which sets standards, and the conscience, which punishes the person for not meeting those standards. In Anthetic Therapy, the concept of the Inner Critic is similar: The "shoulds" are the standards (ego ideal), which are imposed by the Inner Critic (the punitive conscience). Most classical psychoanalysts maintain that the superego emerges from the Oedipus complex and can be loving as well as punitive (Schafer, 1960); therefore addressing the superego, while important, is not the central factor in overcoming personal problems. When the superego is addressed, its harshness should be moderated. In contrast, Anthetic Psychology holds that although the Oedipus complex is an important determinant of Inner Critic functioning, it is not the only one; there are also pre- and post-oedipal determinants. If the Inner Critic is loving, it is so only when the individual obeys its commands. Addressing the Inner Critic must be the initial and central function of psychotherapy. Finally, the goal of Anthetic Therapy is not simply to reduce the Inner Critic's harshness, but to teach the client the skills necessary to become free from every one of the Inner Critic's shoulds. This is achieved by taking back the rights the Inner Critic has tried to take away. The most important distinction between Anthetic Psychology and classical psychoanalysis is that Anthetic Psychology holds that the Inner Critic is the source of shoulds. If the shoulds are disobeyed, the Inner Critic inflicts emotional punishments. This concept is not found in psychoanalysis (or any other school of therapy to date). Writers who mention the Inner Critic (e.g., Paul, 1970) or its analog (e.g., the Voice, Firestone & Catlett, 1999) have understood its ability to criticize but not its ability to impose shoulds and inflict emotional punishments, a process that James E. Elliott (1992b) discovered by analyzing the Anthetic Dialogue sessions of his clients.

Central in Anthetic Psychology is the role of shoulds, a concept influenced by the work of Horney (1950), who maintained that neurosis results from the "tyranny of the should." She further held that shoulds drive the person to actualize an idealized self-image. She saw the goal of therapy as helping to release individuals from the power of shoulds and the illusions of the idealized self, whereupon the real self can emerge. Anthetic Psychology agrees with this formulation and adds items not found in Horney's work, including the concept of the Inner Critic as the source of the shoulds, the emotional punishments that are inflicted when the shoulds are disobeyed, and the technique of making releasing statements.

Anthetic Psychology holds that the origin of Inner Critic shoulds and related emotional punishments is a complex process idiosyncratic to the individual. Unlike Dialectical Behavior Therapy that holds guilt and shame as resulting from invalidating environments (parents, primarily) (Linehan, 1987), Anthetic Psychology offers the concept of prototypes, which includes not only parents, but also relatives, teachers, religious authorities, literature, media, and cultural mythology (Elliott & Elliott, 2000).

While Anthetic Psychology's Inner Critic is comparable to Fairbairn's (1952) internal saboteur or antilibidinal ego, Anthetic Psychology sees the Inner Critic as the source of antilibidinal commands; it further sees the Inner Critic as the source of all shoulds and shouldn'ts, including those concerning any drive, wish, need, emotion, or behavior. For example, one person may have Inner Critic shoulds to exercise personal power, while another has shoulds to never exercise personal power. Also, one person may have Inner Critic shoulds to be tender, while another has shoulds to be tough. In other words, the subject of Inner Critic injunctions may vary from person to person and may contain prohibitions against any and all thoughts, feelings, and behaviors.

Anthetic Psychology views internalization of material in the Inner Critic as motivated by fear of the emotional punishments of defectiveness, guilt, shame, inferiority, and loss of the prototype's love. This fear leads to the learning of shoulds. Anthetic Psychology differs from Fairbairn's view that internalization of rejecting objects is the single source of internal saboteur contents. Anthetic Psychology offers three additional sources (Elliott, K., 1999). One is the child's interpretation of innocuous events. For example, an only child whose mother has given birth to a second child concludes, "I must not have been good enough if she had to have another child." The second source is the child's autonomous production of negative beliefs not originating in a negative introject. For example, children who have received little or no guidance may create a great many imperative shoulds for themselves in order to provide a sense of structure. Third, is the child's inferential overgeneralization of positive reinforcement. For example, a child who has been told by the parent, "Daddy and I are so proud of you that you shared your toys with your cousins" may then develop an Inner Critic should to always share possessions.

Furthermore, in regard to internalization, Anthetic Psychology differs from Fairbairn's view that the rejecting object is an unacceptable aspect of the parent. Instead, Anthetic Psychology holds that what is usually internalized are the Inner Critic shoulds and shouldn'ts that occur in response to the verbal and nonverbal messages of parents and other significant figures.

An important caveat in the process of internalization relates to the role of trauma in the development of both the personality and the person's capacity for relationships. A number of theories view trauma as the source of dysfunctionality. Yet correlational research studies have failed to reveal one-to-one relationships between trauma and emotional problems (Elliott, K., 1999). Rather, a number of theories address intervening variables in the development of dysfunction following trauma. These include classical conditioning (Becker & Skinner, 1983); a reduced sense of self-efficacy (Finkelhor & Browne, 1985; Lindberg & Distad, 1985); and the activation of prior schemata following trauma (e.g., rape) (Frank & Stewart, 1984; Resick & Schnicke, 1992). One important variable on which a number of writers occur is the role of self-blame in the negative effects of trauma (Briere, 1992; Feinauer & Stuart, 1996; Westerlund, 1992). Anthetic Psychology proposes that it is not the trauma per se that causes dysfunction. Rather, it is the learning that one takes from the trauma that creates dysfunction. Dysfunctional learning consists of traumatic commands (Inner Critic shoulds) supported by fear. Therefore, it is the Inner Critic that plays a key role in a person's adjustment following trauma.

Consider the case of John, a 22-year-old graduate student, who consulted the therapist for anxiety about traveling outside the state boundaries of California. Through Anthetic Dialogue (to be described later in this chapter) John remembered that when he was a child, his mother had told him, "Now, don't leave your front yard." In John's mind, this command, along with others like it, became generalized to "Don't leave the safety of home; don't take any risks. Don't have girlfriends. Do things with the family. And don't think about leaving home and getting married." He realized that he had believed and obeyed these injunctions and that they had become the guiding principles of his life. They also had led to vulnerability to anxiety when faced with any opportunity counter to the injunctions. He then understood that his anxiety was not the result of trauma per se, but was a result of dysfunctional learning, caused by traumatic commands and supported by fear.

The commands had become integrated into his Inner Critic, where they continued to program him not to venture from familiar surroundings and not to dismantle his attachment to his mother. This structure stymied the normal individuation that would have empowered him to achieve adult goals. As therapy progressed, John unearthed the dysfunctional beliefs he had learned and challenged them using Anthetic releasing statements. He was able to leave home, find an apartment, and begin to establish a life separate from his family. He eventually began a relationship with a woman and ultimately married her.

While many dysfunctional learnings result from traumatic experiences, most come from parental judgmentalism, anger, and injunctions to remain attached to the family. Anthetic Psychology holds that each dysfunctionality, whether evidenced in cognitions, emotions, behaviors, or somatic stress, is the result of learning.

To elaborate, the Anthetic Psychology understanding of the dysfunctionality sequence follows five steps:

1. Dysfunctional learning. The earlier such learning occurs, the more likely it will be experienced as ego-syntonic and comfortable to the person. The person will describe such dysfunctionality as, "That's just the way I am" or "Without it, I wouldn't be me." In other words, the person normalizes the dysfunction, describing it to the self as normal, legitimate, justified, functional, and "not to be tampered with or changed." Examples include injunctions to "Be tough and domineering"; "Be self-sufficient"; and "Be self-effacing."
2. Wounding. The dysfunctional learning may be triggered and held in place by emotional wounding produced when the person has been the target of anger, judgmentalism, abandonment, neglect, and lack of love and affection. The person may then have unconsciously decided to cope with the pain of the wounding by adopting one of the dysfunctional beliefs listed in the preceding paragraph.
3. Bracketing and challenging. Recovery from the learned dysfunction becomes possible when the person, either through life experiences or in therapy, begins to wonder whether a belief may be contributing to problems one is experiencing. Then follows bracketing that belief, temporarily converting it from an unchallengeable certainty to a provisional hypothesis. At such a point, the person, either spontaneously or with the help of the therapist, may now evaluate it in terms of its constructive or destructive impact on functioning.
4. Post-evaluation. Once evaluated, the learning may be accepted and reinstated or may be seen to be dysfunctional, whereupon it can be placed in a mental category labeled as "inactive; to be unlearned."
5. After unlearning. Without the dysfunctional learning, a vacuum occurs. The individual may feel some discomfort at the loss of a cognitive-emotional structure that heretofore had organized his or her functioning. The therapist must now help the person learn new and more optimal values, principles, and beliefs. This process of unlearning followed by learning is at the heart of Anthetic Therapy. It becomes the core process for resolving any reactive conflict that occurs in the HVR, because reactive conflicts have their source in dysfunctional learning.

Anthetic Therapy

Anthetic Therapy offers a psychotherapeutic approach applying the principles of Anthetic Psychology to human problems. The goal of Anthetic Therapy is to assist persons to gain freedom from reactivity in order that submerged elements of the natural self may emerge into consciousness where they can be integrated, thus making possible more emotional, behavioral, and relational options (Elliott & Elliott, 2000). For example, if the individual holds Inner Critic shoulds that denigrate tender or loving feelings as weak and "cheesy," Anthetic Therapy challenging methods will help the person shift perspective to see their loving emotions as normal and natural and to feel free to choose to express those feelings in words, love notes, or affection.

During therapy, the process of Anthetic growth moves progressively forward in three stages (Elliott & Elliott, 2000):

Stage I, Submergence: Elements in the individual's inner world become disowned and submerged because they have been pejoritized by the Inner Critic. The individual is unaware of these elements, although certain clues in the person's puzzling problems that bring them to therapy point to their existence. Because certain elements are submerged, they are no longer available to the person as options. This stage includes once-conscious elements which have been repressed, together with submerged elements that have never been conscious.

Stage II, Emergence: Elements have begun to emerge and are being integrated into consciousness. They can now be owned and accepted as Anthetic challenging has removed the pejorative overlay from them. The individual becomes free to choose whether or not to actualize these elements.

Stage III, Actualization: Stage II elements, formerly merely in consciousness, may now become actualized in behavior through conscious choice.

An important method used in Anthetic Therapy is Anthetic Dialogue (Elliott, 1992b). An adaptation of the Gestalt empty chair method, Anthetic dialogue has been found useful in eliciting and challenging the negative messages of the Inner Critic. Anthetic Dialogue differs from conventional empty chair work in that it does not rely on back-and-forth dialogue between two chairs in order to resolve the split (Perls, 1969, p. 19) nor to achieve integration (Corey, 1991, p. 250) but instead uses as many chairs as needed to explore phenomenologically inner material such as the Inner Critic, inner figures, and prototypes. Rather the goal is to elicit and challenge dysfunctional beliefs, not integrate them into the personality; to no longer believe Inner Critic messages, not to "soften" or change the Inner Critic (Greenberg, Safran, & Rice, 1989), and to increase options through inner freedom from Inner Critic oppression.

As submerged material begins to emerge through Anthetic Dialogue, the therapist guides the person in Anthetic processing. This procedure involves identifying and challenging Inner Critic injunctions, orchestrating Inner Figures, identifying polar type rigidities, and individuation from prototype influences.

Anthetic Relationship Therapy

Central to Anthetic Relationship Therapy (ART) is the tenet that relationships, particularly intimate ones, provide a primary opportunity for growth for the partners. This perspective is consistent with the theory and research of Aron and Aron's (1997) self-expansion model, which holds that the desire for self-expansion (cognitively, socially, self-conceptually) is a fundamental human motive and that close relationships are key opportunities for expansion to occur. Self-expansion model posits that close relationships offer fundamental fulfillment as each partner includes in the self the other partner's resources, perspectives, and identities (Aron, & Aron, 1986; Aron, Aron, & Norman, 2001; Aron, Mashek, & Aron, 2004). In ART, as partners choose and learn skills for greater voltage (i.e., deeper emotional closeness), growth of each partner occurs.

Anthetic Relationship Therapy offers the concept of inclusive growth, in which all elements in the individual's psyche become accepted for inclusion in the personality. These include emotions, such as anger and hurt feelings, as well as all thoughts, desires, and impulses. ART adds that inclusive growth merely means total self-acceptance as a goal, and that actualizing any element in behavior becomes a choice the person can then make informed by values and principles.

A second prong of growth obtainable through closeness involves maintaining one's individuality while achieving closeness, referred to as intimacy regulation (Prager & Roberts, 2004). ART offers a three-step conceptualization of this process:

1. Fusion: Initially, both developmentally and throughout the life span, the individual is fused both intrapsychically and interpersonally. Intrapsychically, fusions occur as the individual becomes psychologically welded to any number of mental elements. Examples include inner figures, concepts, defensive strategies, and philosophies of life. In the case of a conceptual fusion, the person holds two ideas that do not logically belong together, as in "If someone is angry at me, then I am guilty." Interpersonally, a person may become fused or welded to another person such as a parent or to an organization such as a religious institution or a sports team. When fused interpersonally, the individual does not differentiate self from other.
2. Disengagement: In this step, the individual gains psychological space between the self and any internal element or external entity. From this disengaged position, the person can assess the usefulness or desirability of any given element on the basis of criteria the person has developed. Examples of criteria include values and guiding concepts.

3. Flexible Merging: Once disengaged, the person is free to merge with the element as little or as fully as desired. The concept of flexible merging is central to high-voltage relating. As partners identify a desire for closeness, they may enter such merging as oneness, having learned that they possess skills for disengaging as they choose.

The challenge of intimacy regulation magnifies when the couple have disparate intimacy and autonomy desires (Prager & Roberts, 2004). The Voltage model offers therapists a concept for assisting partners in articulating their intimacy and autonomy desires, as well as for providing skills for navigating voltage desire fulfillment.

Anthetic Relationship Therapy is a skills-based approach, focusing on providing partners skills they can use to clear away dysfunctional learning and internal blocks to intimacy. The intrapersonal and interpersonal skills taught to the couple are intentionally portable, that is, usable outside the therapy session in the couple's ordinary lives.

Also fundamental to ART is the concept that *inner freedom* is necessary for optimal relating (Green, Elliott, & Myrick, 2014). Partners learn skills for neutralizing the Inner Critic, for becoming free from prototype influences, and for gaining polar type flexibility, along with interpersonal skills for creating closeness and resolving conflict. These skills will be covered in later chapters of this book.

As Elliott and Elliott explored using interventional experiments with groups as well as couples, an important benefit of increasing inner freedom emerged. When participants learned to use the skills of Anthetic processing (i.e., Anthetic Dialogue, Inner Critic challenging, and Inner Figure orchestration), they began to unblock warm feelings toward each other. These warm feelings evidenced themselves as distinct from reactive loving feelings in that they were felt and/or expressed simply because they felt good, not because they required reciprocity. The warm feelings became labeled as Anthetic love, love felt and expressed unconditionally, and with no expectation of return (Elliott & Elliott, 2000).

Chapter 3

The Inner Critic and Its Sabotaging Effects on Relationships

Primary reasons couples seek counseling are for communication issues and lack of affection (Doss, Simpson, & Christensen, 2004; Kugel, 2010). As the therapist assists the couple in unearthing the source of such issues, major themes emerge, including schemata for dealing with internal expectations about relationships (Earley, 2012; Epstein & Baucom, 2002; Stinckens, Lietaer, & Leijssen, 2013). Underlying such schemata is an internal construct called the Inner Critic (Green, Elliott, & Myrick, 2014). Its presence and power in psychological functioning has been well documented in the literature from its seemingly earliest mention by Louis Paul (1970). Intimations of the Inner Critic, however, appeared as early as Freud's (1923) discussion of the superego; Perls' (1969) referral to the top dog; and Transactional Analysis references to the Critical Parent (Dusay, 1977).

The Inner Critic is an internal voice that might well be called the Inner Saboteur (Vorhaus, 1966), because it does much more than criticize. Referred to as "the voice" by Firestone & Firestone (2004), it is the composite of introjected destructive thoughts from parents. Anthetic Therapy expands the source of introjected messages to include all negative prototypes, whether parents, teachers, religious authorities, or society. The Inner Critic disrupts intimacy and causes couple distress by creating "drivers," which, when obeyed, result in a driven way of life. The way of life is characterized by partners' reacting compulsively and mechanically, although partners often remain unaware of it. In fact, partners report that such mechanical reactions feel "normal," "natural," "proper," and "appropriate."

The drivers generated by each partner's Inner Critic surface in the clinical process as "shoulds" and "shouldn'ts," of which partners remain mostly unaware (Elliott, 1991; Elliott & Elliott, 2000). The net result is that each partner functions interpersonally in a constricted manner. This constriction results through the Inner Critic's threats to inflict one or more of five

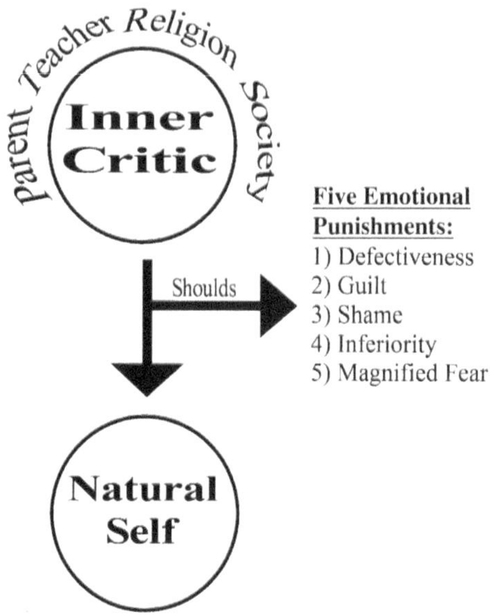
Parent Teacher Religion Society
Inner Critic
Shoulds
Five Emotional Punishments:
1) Defectiveness
2) Guilt
3) Shame
4) Inferiority
5) Magnified Fear
Natural Self

Figure 3.1 Inner Critic Diagram

emotional punishments: feelings of defectiveness, inferiority, guilt, shame, and anxiety (or magnified fear). To illustrate the structure of Inner Critic functioning, see Figure 3.1.

Each time a partner feels a twinge (or jolt) of one of these five punishments, the Inner Critic is the source of each twinge, subconsciously attempting to control the partner. The force of this process becomes evident in a partner reporting that simply *thinking* about disobeying a should results in their feeling one or more of the emotional punishments.

When this process is explained to couples, they often ask, "Isn't the guilt I'm feeling just part of my conscience?" The Anthetic therapist's response is that the conscience is a concept that has held implicit values. The *negative* conscience guides through emotional punishments and is synonymous with the Inner Critic. In contrast, the *positive* conscience offers loving, non-punitive guidance. In ART, the positive conscience is called the Inner Guide. Guidance via the Inner Critic blocks creativity, love, and vitality. Guidance sourced by the Inner Guide engenders creativity, love, and vitality.

In other words, the shoulds and shouldn'ts that comprise the drivers are more than mere rules for living that an individual can easily decide to ignore. These injunctions are powerful commands backed by threats of painful punishment if the individual disobeys them or even thinks about disobeying them.

An interesting complication of this negative guidance process is that individuals may never feel the punishments, because they never think seriously about disobeying the should or shouldn't given the force of the emotional pain threatened to be inflicted if they were to disobey. Consequently, they never stray from the rigid blueprint imposed by the Inner Critic.

Evolutionary explanations have been offered by neuroscientists (Ito, Larsen, Smith, & Cacioppo, 1998), referring to the brain's negativity bias. As human neurobiology has evolved to support survival, the brain's bias to interpret events in a negative light can be seen as an attempt to ensure safety. Thus the Inner Critic comprises the negative messages aimed at keeping the individual safe. However, this safety purpose expands to keeping a person safe from what the Inner Critic perceives as dangers in becoming an autonomous, free, individuated human being. The result is constriction of a person's options (Elliott, K. 1995; Elliott & Elliott, 2000).

The Inner Critic, Decompensation, and Its Impact on Ability to Love

Partners often lament to the therapist, "Why can't we just love each other?" One essential answer lies in the role of the Inner Critic in decompensation. ART offers an explanation of the psychodynamic structure underlying decompensation. A review of Inner Critic function provides the elements through which a therapist can gain understanding of the mechanism of decompensation in partners.

First, the Inner Critic imposes shoulds backed by emotional punishments. The pain of the emotional punishments or their threat is so intense, the partners resort to compensation in the form of buffers (Elliott, 1992b). Buffers include such items as being a good cook; providing ample income to support one's family, and having well-behaved children. As long as partners' buffers are in place, each can remain compensated sufficiently to express love. This structure however has a fundamental vulnerability to failure. Intimate relationships provide myriad opportunities for partners' buffers to collapse. For example, a partner whose buffer consisted of having a good job may lose the job resulting in decompensation. Or a partner whose body was in excellent shape may lose shape during pregnancy, thus resulting in decompensation. In each case, failure of the buffer opens the psychological door to Inner Critic emotional pain in the form of feelings of defectiveness, shame, inferiority and magnified fear. In the face of such pain, partners may resort to defensive maneuvers.

How to Identify if the Inner Critic is Poised to Sabotage a Couple's Relationship

Defensive maneuvers in the decompensated couple appear as symptoms with which the couple presents in therapy. ART has delineated a list of symptoms for which the therapist may watch in a couple in whom Inner Critic functioning is poised to sabotage their relationship. Each symptom is a clue to deeper subconscious machinery that must be dismantled in order that the couple may enjoy an optimal HVR.

1. Negativity. Negativity includes anger, judgmentalism, harshness, vengefulness, and distancing. According to Gottman's (1999) research such negativity is a reliable predictor of not only unhappiness in a marriage but also of divorce. In ART, not only does the therapist identify such negativity but also conceptualizes such corrosive elements as caused directly or indirectly by partners' Inner Critic.
2. Victim Feelings. Feelings of having no free choice have been found to prevent change (Gottman, 1999). Such messages as "This is just the way I am; I can't help it" have their source in the Inner Critic.
3. Touchiness. While touchiness, that is, quick defensive responses, in partners may appear to be simple reactions to what the other partner has said, it can be more than a reaction. It usually is teleological. In ART, touchiness is found to have a functional purpose, of which partners may not be immediately aware. In clinical experience with couples, the goal of touchiness has been found to relate to Inner Critic functioning. When one partner communicates in a way that triggers the other partner's Inner Critic, the triggered partner feels a twinge of emotional pain in the form of one of the five emotional punishments. In order to allay the pain, the person triggered uses the defense of a touchy response. Common touchy responses include anger, biting sarcasm, *tu quo que* comments ("You do it too"), and denial. The purpose of such comments is to intimidate the initiating partner to stop talking and thus stop triggering the Inner Critic. In order to create an HVR, the therapist must help the partners become aware of the purpose of the touchiness. This psychoeducation intervention involves labeling the defensive response with the term *touchiness* followed by a *pull report.* A pull report is a communication that reports an impulse paired with a declaration to not behave in a way consistent with the impulse. The therapist teaches the partners the two-step process: 1. Label the defensive feeling or comment as "Hmm. I'm feeling touchy." 2. Report the pull by stating, "I have a pull to be touchy, but I'm not going to go there."
4. Quotidian Dishonesty. In a standard relationship, quotidian dishonesty is often the primary coping strategy a person in a relationship employs with a touchy partner. The dishonesty has as its purpose to not tell the truth in order to avoid upsetting the partner. Typical Inner Critic messages that fuel this strategy include such thoughts as, "Don't say what you're thinking or feeling. It will only make them mad"; and "If you say what you're feeling, you'll upset your partner." Such messages comprise the shoulds, "You should never make your partner mad. You should never

upset your partner." These shoulds are then backed with the threat of the emotional punishments of guilt, shame, and magnified fear. While this strategy may prevent arguments engendered by touchiness, it comes at the price of closeness.

5. Distancing. As partners choose not to express quotidian thoughts and feelings in an honest and forthcoming manner, distance results. Emotional closeness is the casualty of this strategy commanded by the Inner Critic. In effect, the partners begin to lower the voltage of previous closeness they may have shared.
6. Depression. Psychodynamic taxonomies of depression offer a useful approach to understanding Inner Critic connections to depression. As partners begin to function in their relationship by the strategies of touchiness and dishonesty prescribed by the Inner Critic, they may begin to experience anaclitic depression (Blatt, 1974), the type of depression caused by lack of emotional closeness. In addition, because the Inner Critic delivers injunctions that forbid pleasure, and because partners often obey such injunctions, they experience antihedonic depression. Moreover, because the Inner Critic condemns partners, introjective depression is produced.
7. Beliefs held by partners that they need not learn special skills for creating a satisfying relationship. A common dysfunctional belief held by many partners involves the misconception that they already possess the knowledge to effectively communicate in order to have happiness in their relationships. These beliefs, like other protective messages, have their source in the Inner Critic.
8. The Pursuer-Distancer Pattern. Christensen & Heavey (1993) have identified a common pattern in couples identified as the Pursuer-Distancer pattern (also as the Demand-Withdraw pattern). This pattern is marked by one partner's seeking connection by pursuing, while the other distances or withdraws when pursued. In ART, the Inner Critic has been discovered to command the disparate roles in each partner.
9. Responsibility Tangles. An important and frequent source of arguments in couples occurs when partners believe there are responsible for any negative feelings each might have. This belief creates *responsibility tangles,* marked by accusations by each partner that the other has *made* them angry, humiliated, upset, sad, or fearful. What partners do not realize is that the Inner Critic is the subconscious source of any such feelings. Humiliation, guilt, defectiveness, and fear are direct emotional punishments delivered by the Inner Critic. The partner is merely the trigger for the Inner Critic inflicting such punishments. Anger is the defensive abreaction secondary to feelings of constriction prescribed by Inner Critic shoulds. Instead, partners mistakenly target each other with blame for causing painful feelings.

10. Fear of Intimacy. One protective measure the Inner Critic may employ comprises messages that intimacy is dangerous and must be avoided. In such cases, partners may report to the therapist that intimacy makes him or her uncomfortable. Such fear of intimacy is ego-syntonic, indicated when a partner states, "That's just the way I am."
11. Relationship Problems. Totally apart from the issue of their desire for high-voltage relating, partners may report puzzlement that practically all their relationships are unsatisfying or problematic. In each case, the Inner Critic may be functioning in the partner in the form of feelings of defectiveness, shame, inferiority, and magnified fear. The emotional punishments pervade even non-intimate relationships blocking effective relating.
12. The Need for Revenge. In an effort to re-buffer in the face of decompensation, the Inner Critic may prescribe revenge on the partner for having been the source of the decompensating interaction. Revenge involves some form of distorted psychological justice, thus intrapsychically righting the scales by inflicting pain on the "offending" partner.
13. Drugs or Alcohol. In an effort to deal with Inner Critic inflicted emotional pain, partners may not only resort to psychological buffers but also the mood-altering chemical buffers of drugs or alcohol. Such drugs shift the neurochemistry of the brain, prompting a surge of GABA, the neurochemical associated with suppression of message transmission in the brain (Elliott, K., 2006). Initially, this chemical buffer provides pain relief for partners. However, by the time couples seek therapy, this buffer may be causing myriad problems in the couple's relationship.
14. Defensiveness When Given Feedback. Feedback between partners and from the therapist is essential in the creation of an HVR. Decompensation invoked by the Inner Critic can prevent partners from welcoming and processing this feedback. In the face of such decompensation, partners often become oppositional and defensive.
15. Inability to Feel and Express Love. The ideal archetype of HVR proposed by ART is one in which partners learn skills for liberating and expressing feelings of love for anyone. Such expressions may include both verbal and physical expressions, including hugs and saying, "I feel love for you." ART proposes a special definition of love: *Love is warm feelings.* ART distinguishes love from caring behavior and commitment (Elliott, J., & Elliott, K., 2000, Ch. 17). Because the Inner Critic's role is to protect the person, it will restrict the person to loving only people whom the Inner Critic has labeled "correct" or "appropriate": one's life partner, children, or other relatives. It will constrict and deprive the person of the pleasure of feeling and expressing love to anyone outside that circumscribed circle.

Imperative Shoulds and Recipe Shoulds

As therapists recognize the role of Inner Critic shoulds in couples' relationship difficulties, they may be tempted to conclude erroneously that all shoulds must be proscribed from couples' vocabulary. ART offers an important distinction that resolves this dilemma. ART offers the concept of imperative shoulds versus recipe shoulds. Imperative shoulds are defined as Inner Critic shoulds, that is, drivers that are delivered by the Inner Critic. In contrast, recipe shoulds consist of neutral recommendations that do not come from the Inner Critic but simply tell the individual how to do things effectively. An example of a recipe should is, "If you want to be hired for a job, you should be polite in the job interview." The essential distinction is that a recipe should has no self-esteem issue implied in it, as opposed to an imperative (or Inner Critic) should which involves an implication of lowered self-esteem if one does not obey the should. In the case above, an imperative should would me, "If you want to be hired for a job, you better be polite, Stupid!"

Disarming the Inner Critic's Effects on Relationships

In light of the devastating effects the Inner Critic has on partners and their ability to create closeness, optimal HVRs are predicated upon partners gaining proficiency in skills for disarming the Inner Critic. This disarming process begins with Clue Work. First, the therapist teaches each partner how to uncover drivers, that is, shoulds and shouldn'ts contained in the subconscious mind. One metaphor that has been found useful in explaining this process to couples is that Clue Work to subconscious Inner Critic messages can be discovered just as a person might discover the shape of a hidden magnet by noticing the behavior of certain clues (iron filings) on a sheet of paper. Cognitive and behavioral clues such as touchiness, fear, and the other thirteen items listed above are akin to the iron filings in the metaphor. Just as the iron filings are being affected by the unseen force of the magnet beneath the paper, so also are one's thoughts and behaviors affected and even driven by the unseen force of the Inner Critic. The second step in Clue Work is to teach partners to challenge each Inner Critic should or shouldn't.

Once partners have learned to identify Inner Critic shoulds through Clue work, the second step is to learn to challenge each Inner Critic should or shouldn't; that is, each driver. The goal of ART is to equip partners to use Inner Critic challenging skills on their own. The therapist leads partners through Anthetic Dialogue in which each partner reveals Inner Critic shoulds then challenges the shoulds using releasing statements (Elliott, J.E., 1994; Elliott, J., & Elliott, K., 2000). These releasing statements equip each partner to become free from the reactive rigidity that produces the driven and constricted state of mind underlying couple conflict.

The Emergence of the Natural Self

As partners begin to use releasing statements, they experience increasing freedom from the Inner Critic. As freedom increases, each partner reports what to them is a surprising occurrence, that is, a renewed sense of vitality, a relaxation of tension, and a liberation of love. These events mark what in Anthetic Therapy is termed *the emergence of the Natural Self.* The importance of this emergence is second only to the achievement of inner freedom in laying the foundation for creating an optimal (i.e., high-voltage) relationship.

The Natural Self is the part of the personality that exists before an individual receives any negative programming. It contains the vital energies of the primary self in addition to the structure of the secondary self, containing the schemas for deploying those energies in the world. The Anthetic concept of the primary self is much like the Freudian concept of primary process, the mode of psychological functioning characterized by an urgency for tension reduction (Elliott, J., & Elliott, K., 2000; Freud, 1900/1955; Freud, 1915/1957). The Anthetic concept of secondary self structure is comparable to the Freudian concept of secondary process, characterized by delay of gratification of needs and wishes in order to match primary self needs to the environment (Elliott, J., & Elliott, K., 2000; Freud, 1915/1957 and 1900/1955).

CASE

Anna and Leonard, ages 58 and 62, married 20 years, sought couple counseling for simmering resentments. The couple was involved in an active social life, often dining with other couples in their homes and reciprocating by hosting those friends in their home. They came to this session following one such weekend dinner in their home. Leonard started the session with a report of the week, "We had our ups and downs. One of the downs happened this weekend when we had friends over to dinner. Anna had spaghetti sauce cooking on the stove. Our guests were going to arrive at 6:00, and they're usually on time. I looked at the clock and saw it was 5:25. I thought, 'We ought to put the water on to boil for the pasta.' But I noticed that Anna was in the bathroom putting on makeup. I started feeling stressed. So, I told her, 'I'm going to start the water boiling, because they're gonna be here soon and you're not going to be ready.'" The topic of Anna's not being ready on time for events and Leonard's impatience with her was the source for repeated arguments for the couple. I asked Anna, "What did you feel at that point?"

Anna was tight-lipped and cast a resentful look at Leonard as she responded. "I felt angry. I had been cooking the spaghetti sauce all afternoon. It was ready. I knew it wouldn't take long for the pasta to cook. I just felt controlled by Leonard once again. What I thought was and what I said was, 'That's it. I quit. After tonight, I'm not doing this anymore. And while I meant 'I'm not cooking for company; not entertaining anymore,' I also felt, 'I'm not doing this marriage anymore.'" Leonard voiced surprise. "I hadn't picked up on that last one. I'm glad I didn't."

In conceptualizing this conflict from an Anthetic Relationship Therapy perspective, the couple's discord offers numerous Inner Critic implications. Because Anthetic Relationship Therapy includes psychoeducation of the couple, the therapist offered the elements of the conceptualization to the couple.

She said, "I want to help you see how your Inner Critic was involved in this conflict. I see the love you have for each other and the lovely intention you had to have a nice evening with friends. However, your Inner Critic intervened and sabotaged what could have been a more pleasurable evening for you. Once you identify the Inner Critic's role in this situation, you can then use skills to challenge its messages and get free. Once free from your Inner Critic, you can address the issue in a neutral, even loving way." The couple agreed that they would like that outcome.

The therapist continued, "Leonard, your stress is a clue that your Inner Critic was functioning. Your nervousness contained Inner Critic predictions of disaster that triggered nervousness in you. Can you see what your Inner Critic was predicting?"

Leonard thought for a moment and said, "Hmm, yes, I think it was saying, 'When company is expected; when you've invited them for a certain time, you should be ready 15 minutes beforehand. That's courtesy."

The therapist noted, "So, the Inner Critic was saying, 'You should be ready 15 minutes early or you're being discourteous." Leonard affirmed, "Yes."

Then the therapist offered an important distinction particular to Anthetic Therapy. "I want to help you see an important point about Inner Critic shoulds, so you can be aware of when your Inner Critic is functioning. An Inner Critic should is always an imperative should prescribing what you must do in order to meet the Inner Critic's standards for being 'a worthy person.' If you don't obey the should, your Inner Critic will inflict one or more of the five emotional punishments we've talked about before.

"A recipe should on the other hand, is one that tells you what to do in order to achieve a certain result. For example, 'If you want to bake a good cake, you should use two eggs.' There is no issue of self-esteem involved. If a recipe should is not obeyed, there is no psychological pain. Your psychological pain, Leonard, was in the form of nervousness (magnified fear); a certain clue that your Inner Critic was pouncing."

Leonard nodded. "I hadn't seen that. That's helpful."

The therapist continued. "One more way your Inner Critic increased your stress was by tying a should to be ready 15 minutes early to a value you hold; that of being courteous. What the Inner Critic did is called a *fusion*. A fusion is when one fuses or welds together two ideas that do not logically belong together. The Inner Critic said that to be anything but 15 minutes early is to be discourteous. Can you see that way of thinking as placing the attitude of courtesy on an arbitrary timeline created by the Inner Critic? Your courtesy toward your guests is not logically connected to that timeline." Here the therapist is explaining in layman's terms the concept of *defusing conceptual fusions* (Elliott, J.E., 1991; Elliott, J., & Elliott, K., 2000).

The therapist then taught the couple the Inner Critic challenging skill of the "Just Because" technique (Elliott, J.E., 1991). "In order to defuse the fusion, you can use the 'Just Because' technique. In this case, you can say to your Inner Critic, 'Just because I'm not ready 15 minutes early does not make me discourteous.'" Leonard said this statement out loud and said he saw the logic of it.

Additionally, in order to strengthen Leonard's movement toward inner freedom, the therapist taught Leonard the *What You Call* technique (Elliott, J., & Elliott, K., 2000). "Whenever the Inner Critic gives you a pejorative message that puts you down (as it did when it implied you were being discourteous), you can say to it, 'I have the right to be *what you call* discourteous.' This will release you from buying into the bullying message from the Inner Critic by exposing that its message is not valid; merely name-calling." Leonard then tried the statement out loud, "I have the right to be *what you call* discourteous." He said it while nodding and followed with, "That feels right; better."

Once the therapist had helped Leonard identify and dismantle the structure of his stress that had contributed to the conflict, she turned to Anna and said, "Anna, let's see how the Inner Critic was functioning in you in this conflict. When Leonard said, 'You're not going to be ready,' you said you felt controlled." (Anna nods.) "There is a subtle imperative should implied here, and it is, 'You shouldn't be controlled.'"

(Anna says with surprise, "Yes!")

The therapist continues, "Now this has power, because the Inner Critic is adding an emotional punishment to the concept of 'being controlled.' Can you tell what follows after, 'You shouldn't be controlled, because if you're controlled, you're ________'?"

Anna thought a moment and added, "If you're controlled then you're one-down."

The therapist expanded, "So, being one-down is the emotional punishment of inferiority, which feels psychologically painful."

Anna agrees, "Oh, yes!"

The therapist asks, "Can you see that your Inner Critic was pouncing on you and making you feel very bad in response to Leonard's comment?"

Anna unhesitatingly replies, "Yes, I do!"

Realizing that an important explanation was necessary here, the therapist continued, "Now, I want to point out probably the most important reason why Inner Critic work is essential for reducing your conflict. Because your Inner Critic is making you both feel emotional pain, you, of course, want relief from the pain. Seeking pain relief is, of course, a natural response in us humans to pain. When the pain has its source in the Inner Critic, as partners, we try a number of ways to get free from the pain. One of them is what happened with you, Leonard. Your Inner Critic criticized you with the message that you were being discourteous and paired that criticism with the emotional pain of guilt. You did a common response to that pain by turning it outward onto Anna through criticizing her."

As the therapist explained, Leonard began nodding his head in recognition and agreement.

The therapist continued, "Anna, as Leonard criticized you, your Inner Critic inflicted the emotional pain of defectiveness ('You're late') and inferiority ('You're being controlled'; that is, one-down)." (Anna nods.) "In the face of that pain, you sought relief through a common strategy that partners use—giving up ('That's it. I quit.')."

Anna laughs and says, "Yes, that explains it!"

Summarizing the strategy the couple can use in the future for such conflict, the therapist offers, "I want to suggest two steps for you both to use in order to protect your relationship from your Inner Critic. In step one, realize any tension or pain you feel is first and foremost between you and your Inner Critic. This will be essential in shifting you from automatically thinking it's about you and your partner. For you, Leonard, when you feel tense or stressed and feel the impulse to criticize Anna, label these feelings, 'That's my Inner Critic.' In step two, Leonard, I recommend you tell Anna, 'I think my Inner Critic is pouncing since I wanted to criticize you for not getting ready. But I'm not going to do it.'"

"Anna, when you feel like saying, 'That's it. I quit,' I recommend you label that thought, 'That's my Inner Critic.' Then turn to Leonard and say, 'Leonard, I think my Inner Critic is pouncing because I want to tell you, 'That's it,' but I'm not going to go there.'"

An analysis of the Anthetic Therapy Process in this case reveals three major points particular to Anthetic Relationship Therapy. First, the therapist is alert to the intervening variable of the Inner Critic in all couple conflict. This dynamic is akin to the Internal Family Systems Therapy concept of parts (Schwartz, 1995). As Schwartz noted, identifying the intervening variable helps couples shift out of an adversarial position with each other and instead to be free to relate. However, ART not only introduces the couple to the role of the Inner Critic as adversary inciting the conflict but also describes the dynamic of shoulds and emotional punishments inflicted by the Inner Critic. Second, the ART therapist teaches the couple skills to employ to become free from Inner Critic messages. Third, ART encourages the couple to become allies in identifying and getting free from the Inner Critic.

Understanding Defensiveness: Defensive Ploys

Defensiveness in couples may trigger anxiety in the therapist as well as each partner. The Anthetic Relationship Therapy archeology of defensiveness can help the therapist and partners understand the structure of defensiveness. Under the barrage of Inner Critic messages triggered by intimate relating, each partner decompensates producing in each what ART labels the Devalued Self. This internal structure is marked by feelings of defectiveness, shame, inferiority, guity, and anxiety (i.e., the five emotional punishments). In response, subconscious processes for compensating for the pain of the Devalued Self produce the Buffering Self, which comprises the buffers found useful during the partner's lifetime for pain relief. The Devalued Self together with the Buffering Self comprise each partner's Reactive Self; the self each mistakenly thinks they are. When partners feel touchy and defensive, it is the Reactive Self that feels touchy and defensive. This system appears ego-syntonic as a result of a fusion of the Natural Self with the Reactive Self. As such, each partner describes their defensive responses as "That's just the way I am." As long as this fusion remains out of conscious awareness of the partners, each will rely on defensive ploys for emotional protection from subconscious Inner Critic-induced pain.

In the intense atmosphere of intimacy, partners are continually giving each other feedback. Such feedback may be communicated in the form of requests for change, complaints about the partner, and critical comments. Each incidence of feedback threatens to disconfirm the Reactive Self, with the concomitant threat of decompensation. To avoid the painful feelings of humiliation, inferiority, and defectiveness, partners resort to defensive ploys. Following is a list consisting of common examples of defensive maneuvers found in clinical practice.

1. Acquittal Statements. Here the person who is the recipient of feedback tries to get acquitted of what is labeled a "crime" by the Inner Critic. For example, in the case of Laura and Richard, Laura states, "You're hardly ever affectionate with me anymore." In response, Richard offers

an automatic acquittal, "I give you plenty of affection. I hug you; I kiss you every time I leave for work." Richard acquittal response, commanded by his Inner Critic, is an example of an attempt to stave off the threatened debuffering he perceives in Laura's request. He will benefit by the therapist asking, "Did you feel a twinge of pain at Laura's statement?" The therapist then offers the label of "Acquittal Statement" to Richard, along with the explanation that acquittal statements are measures commonly used to defend against Inner Critic pain triggered by the partner's feedback. Following this, the therapist would teach the skill of a *Pull Report*. In the instance, the Pull Report would consist of Richard declaring, "I have a pull to try to get acquitted, but I'm not going to go there."

2. Silence. Partners may often deploy a defense of becoming silent. The therapist may assume that the silence could be attributed to inattentiveness or being distracted. However, silence is a frequently used counter-humiliation strategy, that is, a way of evading making a response that would trigger humiliation.
3. Affability. This defense comprises responding to one's partner's feedback with what appears to be common sense, moderation, and restraint.

    ELAYNA: "I feel alone raising the kids. You never help me."

    MARK: "You're making a mountain out of a mole-hill. You don't need to treat kids like hothouse plants. Why not just be more accepting?"

Often the affability defense is spoken with a smile or a chuckle. The calm, amused demeanor may befuddle the partner into doubting the validity of the original request. The therapist helps the couple by asking each partner what feelings occurred when the other spoke. Partners like Mark, who rely on affability to avoid Inner Critic pain, may need help to see that they use subtle judgmentalism to dismiss feedback. The Anthetic Relationship Therapist then helps Mark to use a challenging statement to become free from the Inner Critic. In this case, the therapist taught Mark a Just Because statement: "Just because you feel alone and say I never help you doesn't mean I'm a bad person or have done anything wrong." Once free from Inner Critic pain, Mark is able to consider Elayna's feedback and then address it in a task-oriented way.

4. Switching the Topic. The purpose of the topic switch is to avoid responding to something the partner has just said; hopefully, without the partner noticing. A common variety of topic switch involved making a counter-complaint or cross-complaining. This defense often is successful in avoiding decompensation, because the first partner is so motivated to respond that he or she will abandon the topic initially presented and instead pursue the new topic.

A common example of topic switching is:

WILLIAM: "You don't respect me."

BARBARA: "Well, you don't respect me."

WILLIAM: "Yes, I do."

In this communication, William abandoned his original topic in order to get acquitted of Inner Critic condemnation triggered by Barbara's topic switch. Once the partners understand the concept of the Inner Critic and its functioning, the therapist can intervene by asking Barbara, "Did your Inner Critic pounce when William said you don't respect him?" As Barbara identifies the twinge of emotional pain she felt, she can make a releasing statement using the Just Because technique, "Just Because you tell me I don't respect you doesn't mean I'm a bad person or have done something wrong." Once free from her Inner Critic, Barbara can address in detail and in a neutral way what William is feeling.

5. Following a Justice Script. The Justice Script is a variation on the topic switch in which the partner invokes the principle of justice. For example:

   JENNIFER: "I have a request that you show me more affection."

   BARRY: "Well, isn't this a two-way street? I have a request that you show me more affection."

   While Barry's response may sound reasonable, it actually switches the topic deflecting what Jennifer said through an invocation of the principle of justice. The therapist in this case guided the couple to become free of Inner Critic material contained in the communication by helping Jennifer make a Releasing Statement:

   JENNIFER: "I have the right to ask for more affection, even though *I* don't show more affection."

   The therapist also helped Jennifer make a request of Barry; that is, "I have a request that you respond to my topic first; then I'll respond to yours. Let's take turns."
6. Naturalizing. This defense involves trying to interpret problems not as something from which to recover but rather as "just natural." Examples include, "It's just natural to be angry." "Who wouldn't feel bad in those circumstances?" "It's normal to want your own space a lot." The therapist can guide the partner to reflect that while the problem might be commonly experienced by others, that does not mean that it would not be beneficial to address it as material from which to become free, particularly if it is detrimental to the relationship.
7. Ambiguizing. This defense includes the offering of vague or incomplete information that could be interpreted as positive but which is actually negative. The information a partner offered, while true, is incomplete.

Take the case of Selena, who presented in therapy with deep pain in response to her husband Joe's harsh criticism. After months of her requesting that Joe see a therapist, he at last agreed. He has been to one session on April 5.

Joe has just returned from this first therapy session and has described it to Selena. He stated that he is not sure it helped, but Selena is hopeful.

SELENA: "When is your next appointment?"

JOE: "The 12th."

SELENA (*counting to herself:* next week! She is overjoyed): "Oh, good!"

Joe is silent.

On April 11th, Selena says, "You have your appointment tomorrow." Joe says nothing. Selena is concerned. Ordinarily, Selena would overlook Joe's silence, but this time she asks, "Is that correct?"

JOE: "Is what correct?"

SELENA: "That you have a therapy appointment tomorrow."

JOE: "I didn't say that."

SELENA: "You said the 12th."

JOE: "Well, my appointment is the 12th of July. I'm seeing the therapist every three months."

SELENA: "You lied to me!"

JOE: "No, I didn't. I said the 12th, and that's what it is. Just get the cotton out of your ears, dammit!"

Selena faces a dilemma. Can she be satisfied with Joe attending therapy every three months? She decides not. The next day she offers Joe an ultimatum: "I see now that you weren't lying to me, but you were trying to befuddle me. I want you to see your therapist once a week, and I want you to tell me your progress each week, or we're through. I can't take the pain anymore."

JOE: "You sound like my mother." (Joe employs a topic switch.)

An analysis of Selena and Joe's argument reveals the following:

- When Joe said "the 12th," he was answering honestly, although incompletely. He used ambiguity to defend against an impending Inner Critic attack. He would have experienced Inner Critic pain if he had told the complete truth, because he would have been revealed to have been doing something about which Selena would have been upset. The therapist conceptualizes this dynamic as a common relationship should inflicted by the Inner Critic, "Do Not Upset Your Partner." Moreover, Joe was attempting to avoid the humiliation he would feel for not carrying out his promise of seeing a therapist weekly.

- On April 11th, Joe uses silence as a further defense strategy. In this case, Selena is more aware and is not distracted.
- Selena next makes a focused request. Joe makes an attempt at switching the topic to an accusation, when he says, "You sound like my mother." Selena could respond with an acquittal statement, e.g., "I'm not at all like your mother." Instead, she correctly ignores the switch and makes a releasing statement in order to become free from the Inner Critic message contained in Joe's statement, "You shouldn't be like your mother."
- Joe's subconscious strategies have as their purpose to preserve his buffers and thereby prevent Inner Critic feelings of humiliation.

Anthetic Relationship Therapy at this point involved teaching Joe how to neutralize his Inner Critic so he could non-defensively listen to Selena's feedback. The marriage began moving toward a high-voltage level.

8. Saying "Okay." The word "Okay" is a variation of ambiguity. For example:

RACHEL: "I want us to have a High-Voltage Relationship."

THOMAS: "Okay."

Two weeks later. . .

RACHEL: "Let's try some of the things in this High-Voltage book."

THOMAS: "I don't want to."

RACHEL: "I thought you said you wanted to."

THOMAS: "No. I just said 'Okay.'"

RACHEL: "Well, what did that mean, Okay?"

THOMAS: "It meant 'I hear you.' That's all."

In the ensuing session, the therapist facilitated Anthetic Dialogue with Thomas, which revealed that Thomas's Inner Critic was commanding him not to obligate himself to anything and at the same time, not to upset Rachel. Saying, "Okay," served as a defense against further Inner Critic shoulds to not engage in an HVR of honesty and self-revelation, because his "defectiveness" would be exposed.

9. Defensive Humorizing. Humorizing is a defense involving responding with humor to the partner who has said something serious. For example, Carla, a young wife, was listening to love songs on the radio. She felt a surge of love for her husband. She told him about one of the songs and sang two lines from it: "'I really love you. I'd even buy the east side of heaven if you blinked your eye.' That's how I feel about you."

"Yeah," he replied. "You're always wanting to buy things. Heh-heh."

Carla's husband's response involves decreasing the intensity of Carla's expression of love. Clinical experience reveals that such defenses are attempts by a partner to counter the Inner Critic should to *do* something in response to receiving someone's love. In this case, the therapist helped her husband to see his Inner Critic should and to use the Just Because statement, "Just because you express love doesn't mean I have to do anything." In addition, the therapist explained to him that he could also just enjoy the warm feeling of love and say nothing; say "Thank you"; or just say, "That feels good." He chose to say, "That feels good."

10. Crypticism. Crypticism involves speaking in a cryptic or obscure manner. For example:

LOUIS: "I need some information on baseball."

CYNTHIA: "Delphi."

LOUIS: "I'm sorry. Delphi?"

CYNTHIA: "Yes, Delphi."

Finally, Cynthia reveals that she is referring to an internet source.

Such cryptic comments when analyzed comprise attempts by the partner to obtain a buffer of superiority over the partner, thus inoculating against Inner Critic pain.

11. Disconnecting. The defense of disconnecting includes responding indirectly or tangentially or leaping ahead to a solution or not responding at all. The clearest example occurs when a partner declares, "I don't want to talk about it."

Take the case of Aaron and his partner, Dan, who had not been getting along well. On the day of their anniversary, Dan said he wanted to celebrate with a meal at an expensive restaurant. Aaron said he wanted to visit friends that evening by himself. He acted on that desire by leaving and returning much later.

Dan asked, "Did you think of the possible effect on me when you left to be with your friends?"

Aaron replied, "It wouldn't have mattered what I did, stayed or walked out." Aaron's reply was not a direct response to Dan's question. He instead disconnected.

Dan felt not only the pain of being left alone but also the pain of disconnection.

The therapist helped Dan make a request to not do that anymore, in the process helping Aaron to challenge Inner Critic shoulds to say "yes" to Dan's request. From that free position, Aaron was able to consider what he wanted to do.

A careful review of each of the defenses listed above reveals that each is driven by a command from the partner's Inner Critic. Each defense can be overcome as the therapist assists the partner in challenging the Inner Critic. One useful and global releasing statement the therapist can teach partners who feel tempted to defend is the following Releasing Statement: "I don't have to defend myself." Once partners become free, the Inner Critic's destructive influence on the relationship is neutralized. On the other hand, each, if overlooked, can sabotage the couple's attempts to create a safe haven where high voltage relating can take place.

THE FOUR ANTHETIC POLAR TYPES

While the Inner Critic influences relationships in a number of intrapersonal ways driving partners to relate from defensiveness in order to protect each one's compensatory buffer system, it also is responsible for the creation of a peculiar kind of one-sidedness that leads to severe conflict and dysfunctionality in relationships. The one-sidedness occurs in the form of polar types, each of which comprises another reactive sub-system. This polarity functioning in partners often prevents the couple from relating optimally in order to create a successful HVR.

Although a number of theories offer personality typologies, few connect these types with underlying dynamics. Satir (1964) offers communication style types. Myers-Briggs Type Inventory offers types based on Jungian theory. Emotionally Focused Couple Therapy (2004) refers to partner functioning based on styles from Attachment Theory.

Anthetic Psychology, on the other hand, describes four personality types, each of which has psychodynamic connections to current hidden influences in the subconscious psyche (see Figure 3.2).

Each type is produced by submerging its opposite. Each submergence occurs at the command of the Inner Critic, locked in place by shoulds. If one of the submerged items would threaten to emerge, the person might feel anxiety, for which there would be no conscious (i.e., surface) explanation. Were any elements of the submerged material to actually emerge, the person would feel one of the five emotional punishments: feelings of defectiveness, guilt, shame, inferiority, and/or anxiety. To avoid these feelings, the individual might have a strong interest in maintaining the submergence of disowned elements, totally out of awareness. The result is that the person is only clearly aware of the polar type that is available to consciousness. The conscious polar type is the one that the person has hyper-cultivated. It will exist as a configuration that seems to have been freely chosen but which in reality is driven.

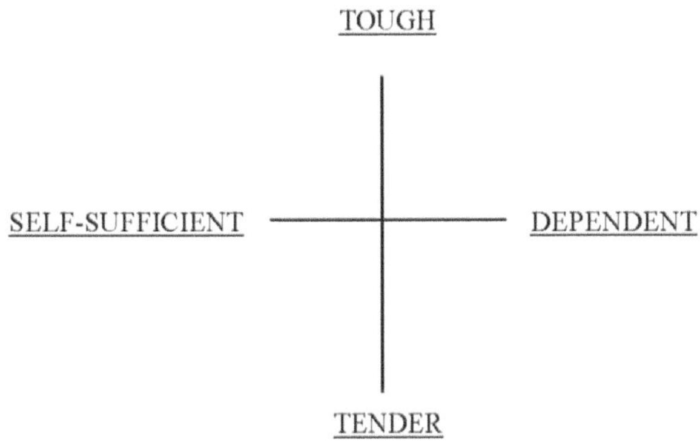

Figure 3.2 Anthetic Polar Types in Relationships

This dynamic offers an explanation for touchiness and defensiveness in the partners. Any touchy or defensive behavior is simply occurring out of fear of the emergence of one or more of the polar elements the person has disowned and submerged. The clinical opportunity arises as the therapist explains this dynamic polar structure and its functioning and offers the partners to work in therapy on bringing the material to awareness.

As partners gain skills for accomplishing the de-submergence of the polar material, executive strength increases. Such strengthening of the executive self equips partners to tolerate the honesty and assertiveness involved in high-voltage relating. Without this strength, the couple will have more difficulty in achieving closeness.

An important caveat in partners' engaging in polar type therapeutic work is that partners may mistakenly do so with the goal of strengthening their one-sidedness. Such work supports the Inner Critic's domination of the partners' lives. A clue to this process is when a partner declares, "I need to get the motivation to do what I know I should be doing." At the same time, the Inner Critic may operate subconsciously to create a cover story to explain and minimize the problems the polarization produces. For example, partners may say, "That's just the way I am" or "If I were to change, I wouldn't be me" or "I don't need therapy; I'm doing okay the way I am, except for this one little thing that seems to be making my relationships unsatisfying. It's probably my partner's fault anyway, not mine."

Upon becoming aware of the connection between conscious polar type and its subconscious cause, partners can take steps to overcome the one-sidedness and thereby enjoy a more flexible personality style while creating a successful HVR.

Following is how the dynamically connected typology works, along with a detailed exploration of the four types:

When a partner submerges one side of the personality and cultivates its opposite, the result is the creation of a polar type which will dominate the personality, that is, Tough, Tender, Self-Sufficient, or Dependent.

Tough people submerge their Tender qualities; Tender people submerge their Tough qualities. Self-Sufficient individuals submerge their Dependent and needy qualities; Dependent individuals submerge either their Tough and/or Self-Sufficient qualities. In each case the personality is impoverished, as submerged qualities are not available for deployment, and options for functioning are diminished.

The Tough Polarity

Individuals who exhibit the Tough polarity consistently live by shoulds to be strong, objective, logical, realistic, and successful. They enjoy competition and a fight of almost any kind, from bar fights to military battles. They often are driven to win at all costs. The driving psychological force behind this is the urge to avoid the humiliation of losing or being inferior that is inflicted by the Inner Critic. They frequently start couple arguments in order to not have to experience that humiliation. Examples can be seen in drivers who may not let a car get ahead of them but must pass car after car until they are ahead of everyone else. Further, if a car enters the freeway in front of them, they construe this as, "He cut me off," and they must get revenge by pulling ahead of the car to undo the humiliation of being "behind." Another way of explaining is that they seek to heal the self-image injury they have suffered by restoring the collapsed buffer of always being first.

In conversations, Tough individuals exhibit competitiveness. If someone mentions having bought a new digital device, the Tough person will talk about *his* device and how superior it is. Tough persons often engage in Experience Matching instead of Interested Questioning, skills to be discussed later in the book. Tough persons find challenges to their knowledge, expertise, or wisdom intolerable. If a Tough person must listen to others, admit ignorance, or learn from others, he or she will feel humiliation at being in an inferior position. The feeling arises from Inner Critic pain resulting from decompensation at being in a one-down position.

Anthetic theory holds that individuals who function rigidly from the Tough pole probably started out life functioning as Tenders. However, during their adolescent development, they realized how much pain they were experiencing as a result of their Tenderness and made a decision for Toughness. They were left with a residual inability to tolerate tenderness and softness. They vocalize that they see these qualities as weak, frivolous, or childish and therefore humiliating. Tough types view others as "contacts" to make and manipulate, not as fellow human beings with whom to empathize and relate to on an equal and mutually involved basis.

An important concomitant of rigid polar type functioning is the tendency to criticize opposite pole functioning. Each pole criticizes in others the qualities that the Inner Critic criticizes in them. This criticalness has significant implications for partner relationships. Tough polar types criticize in their partners any softness, weakness, or tenderness. They do not tolerate crying. In fact, they see their own inability to cry as a virtue.

Tough types are also apt to criticize others for being impulsive, emotional, and irrational. As one husband in therapy said to his wife, "No man wants to listen to all this cryin' and moanin'. Just tell me what the problem is. Let's get down to brass tacks." Tough partners do not like excuses. They feel judgmental toward expressing emotional pain and often label such expressions "whining." The Tough person will also pressure his or her partner to be strong and tough like himself or herself. He or she will have contempt for the partner's dependence and timidity.

Tough people find it easy to exercise personal power. During Anthetic Dialogue they consistently exhibit Inner Critic shoulds not to be cowardly. They hate being dominated or disrespected. As one Tough partner said, "I don't take shit from no one." They enjoy being in command and demand obedience, which, when they get it, serves as a buffer.

During therapy, they have great difficulty doing the Anthetic Listening skill (Chapter 9). They want to offer immediate solutions. As one Tough partner said, "I hate just sitting here while my wife beats about the bush."

An essential difficulty the partner who is a rigid Tough type presents in couple therapy is that obedience to subconscious Inner Critic shoulds to avoid Tenderness culminates in cynicism about love. Such blocks to feeling and expressing love results in relationship difficulties and an inability to create an HVR.

Extreme examples of Tough personalities are Archie Bunker, Adolf Hitler, and Al Capone. They may also be found among military officers, hit men, criminal gang members, some business executives, and terrorists bent on recovering national honor. The psychological process that produces vengeance in a nation is analogous to that which produces vengeance in a marriage. In each instance, the Inner Critic in the Tough person condemns Tenderness and prescribes the Tough compensatory buffer of revenge.

Therapeutic strategies for helping the Tough person involve psychoeducation regarding the Inner Critic's role in rigid polar functioning; Anthetic Dialogue for identifying specific shoulds to be Tough; and challenging techniques for getting free from obeying the shoulds. Therapy consists of challenging the Inner Critic, followed by a radical value shift that permits the addition of Tenderness to the Tough person's repertoire. During this process, the Tough person learns to love.

The Tender Polarity

Individuals who become fused with the Tender polarity function in an opposite manner to Tough persons. They have shoulds to be helpful, sensitive, caring, and emotionally expressive. They value love and closeness and dislike conflict and competition.

The Tender pole is created as Inner Critic shoulds become installed, usually in childhood. The shoulds command the submergence of any inner figures that would want to win and triumph over others. In fact, a Tender person feels guilt if those figures begin to emerge. Moreover, the Tender person's Inner Critic requires that the person identify with the underdog in any conflict automatically and unwittingly. One good example of a Tender person is the character Melanie in the movie *Gone with the Wind.*

The Inner Critic also demands that the Tender person see ordinary assertiveness as rude and aggressive. One consequence of this pattern is a power give-away, in which the person becomes deferential to others. Such power giveaways lead to resentment, anger, and even rage in the Tender individual. This, of course, may not be a conscious process; yet the Tender's partner feels the impact of the usually Tender person's veiled anger.

In intimate relationships, the Tender person exhibits a pattern of behaving in a way to avoid offending others or making them upset. Driven to please the partner and finding it impossible to achieve perfectly, the Tender explodes with puzzling anger. This anger may occur as hatred and may eventuate in the Tender leaving the relationship. "It's the only solution," one Tender wife reported. "I was being tormented beyond my limits. Even if he changes, I wouldn't want to stay with him now."

Couple therapy with the Tender person involves first through Anthetic Dialogue, evoking the person's Inner Critic shoulds, followed by teaching Inner Critic challenging skills.

The Self-Sufficient Polarity

A person who falls into this category has shoulds to be independent, autonomous, and not to need or depend on anyone. The Self-Sufficient person may even welcome the archetypal Self-image of the Lone Wolf. Classic examples of Self-Sufficients are the characters portrayed by Clint Eastwood, John Wayne, and Humphrey Bogart.

In relationships, the Self-Sufficient partner likes to do things without consultation with a partner. When asked questions about themselves, they are apt to give partial answers. The partner of a Self-Sufficient often complains, "Getting a response out of him is like pulling teeth!"

Observation of the development of Self-Sufficients indicates that they often began their lives as Tenders, then because of suffering emotional hurt made early decisions never to open their hearts to anyone again. Uncomfortable with closeness, their behavior became withdrawn, both physically and emotionally. Although they may long for it, closeness seems dangerous to them. They have great difficulty tolerating intimacy, because they fear it, and they fear it because they lack the skills for being Tenderly assertive (and still free) in an intimate relationship. They choose being alone, which is often the only way they can feel totally free. Being Lone Wolves also permits them to avoid conflict, which they hate because of their self-disempowerment.

Not only do they have difficulty in asking for help, they have trouble even admitting they need help. The net result is that they feel comfortable only in an LVR with its style of surface conversations, because in that climate they do not have to deal with conflict.

Self-Sufficients have difficulty asking for directions in a strange city. In fact, they do not like to ask for anything, because, at the command of their Inner Critic, they interpret asking as begging and they would rather go without in order to avoid the humiliation of begging. Any sign of neediness or dependence, they think is a sign of weakness, rather than a perfectly ordinary feeling.

They cannot ask for affection, because it too would be a sign of dreaded neediness. Karl and Marta were married one year and then had a baby. Marta was attending evening classes so she could obtain a better job. Marta's focus on the baby and on classes resulted in Karl feeling left out. However, he was a Self-Sufficient polar type and could not bring himself to complain. His thinking was, "Even if I ask for affection, and she gives it, it won't be given from her desire but because I pleaded with her, and that will just show how weak and valueless I am. It will be humiliating. So I won't say a word." He suffered for years; then suddenly filed for divorce. He had no insight into why he was doing it. He reflected to himself, "I've had enough." His lack of insight left him unable to understand that Self-Sufficiency was the source of his pain. "She should have known I wanted affection without my asking," he said.

Like Tenders, Self-Sufficients may also live by the injunction "Don't try to change your partner." This position disempowers them from making persuasive requests with the result that their needs go unmet. Sooner or later like Karl they often just leave the relationship. Because they have not talked to their partner, the partner may never know why.

As a result of their self-disempowerment, they often complain of feeling pressured, cornered, trapped, and suffocated. However, they are not impervious to feeling lonely, which may lead them to form an intimate relationship.

They may begin the relationship by being close and loving, but at some point they start to feel smothered. At that point they often start arguments over minor issues. Even they are puzzled when they begin to find fault with their partner. For the Self-Sufficient, leaving would trigger guilt; so if complaints can trigger enough dissatisfaction in the partner for them to initiate leaving, the Self-Sufficient avoids guilt.

Self-Sufficient individuals are avoidant of commitment. They are consistent with the Horney style of *Moving Away From (*Horney, 1950) as well as the attachment style of *Avoidant* (Ainsworth, Blehar, Waters, & Wall, 1978). They find commitment constricting and anxiety provoking. Psychodynamically, the reason for the feeling of constrictedness is not in the institution of marriage itself but rather that the Self-Sufficient's Inner Critic disempowers the person from being assertive in relationships.

In therapy, Self-Sufficient individuals are hypersensitive to even the slightest pressure or attempt to influence them. In Anthetic Relationship Therapy, they may accept the partner's request to move toward a more optimal style of relating. However, the process of learning skills needed to achieve that optimality often triggers anxiety, because they feel they will lose their independence. They may view their partners' requests as attempts to control them or be demanding. Likewise, Self-Sufficient partners will view making requests on their own behalf as begging, which their Inner Critic characterizes as demeaning. One person in therapy, Hank, said he did not want to suggest an outing to his partner Jules because, as Hank said, "I didn't want to push myself on him." Whereupon Jules (who was a Tender) said, "Go ahead! Push yourself on me! I want you to take the initiative more." Hank had difficulty believing Jules could really mean it.

Self-Sufficient people often have Tender and Dependent layers just under the surface, and the Self-Sufficient layer serves as a defense against them. Thus the withdrawnness is the Self-Sufficient person's solution to the problem of vulnerability. To put this still another way, Self-Sufficient people use distancing to protect themselves from submitting to the partner's influence. Given their Tender, Dependent tendencies submission is a great temptation for them, so they are on guard much of the time against it. Distancing provides a feeling of safety from any resulting decompensation were they to become close.

Therapy for the Self-Sufficient partner must focus on consistently identifying the person's Inner Critic shoulds to give away their power to their partner ("I have the right to make requests"); to disengage fusions using the Just Because technique ("Just because you make a request does not mean I have to say 'Yes'"); and to become free from accepting the Inner Critic's pejoritizing of neediness as "begging" using the What You Call Technique ("I have the right to do *what you call* begging, Inner Critic"); and the YASNY Technique ("You ain't seen begging till you see what I can do!").

The Dependent Polarity

Emotionally starved, the dependent person will do anything in order to obtain a few crumbs of love and approval. Dependent shoulds include: to be loving and accepting, to be flexible, to be a perfect partner, and to be totally understanding and giving. Dependent types overvalue love and are perfectly willing to disempower themselves in exchange for it. They submerge anger so as to appear super-sweet. An extreme example of the Dependent type is the archetypal victim of abuse, who remains in an abusive relationship for the moments of love the partner gives. If the partner is beginning to individuate in order to become free from enmeshment, the Dependent person will experience severe anxiety.

Whereas Tough persons are hypervigilant about any disobedience that might be displayed by their partners, Self-Sufficients are hypervigilant about being influenced by them. Whereas Tenders are hypervigilant about being criticized, Dependents are hypervigilant about possible rejection and abandonment. The Dependent partner monitors the relationship carefully and takes note of any clues to withdrawal on the part of their partners. If a Dependent's partner is busy working on a project, the Dependent may interpret the situation as one of rejection and abandonment. Dependent types tend to put others in one of two categories: givers and nongivers. The givers are those who will give them the desperately needed emotional supplies of love and approval they crave. If other people refuse to do this, the Dependent will feel hurt, angry, and indignant.

Therapy to assist the Dependent person involves Anthetic Dialogue for identifying the Prototype who was the source of Black Hole pain underlying the Dependent polarization. The identification is supplemented with Anthetic Primal work. Here the therapist facilitates catharsis plus empathic expressions in which the Dependent person offers the Anthetic Sacrament to the Inner Figure who experienced the lack of love and affection that produced the original deprivation.

Pride as a Clue to the Polar Type

Each polar type takes pride in its characteristics. For example, the Tough person is proud of winning. The Tender person is proud of his or her sensitivity, caring, and ability to love. The Self-Sufficient person is proud of her independence. The Dependent person is proud of his independence. The Dependent person is proud of his or her undemandingness, submissiveness, being all-forgiving, and having the ability to adapt.

Such pride is based in the compensatory value of the polar type's characteristics. While the Inner Critic convinces each person of his or her defectiveness, the buffers contained in each type's functioning becomes highly valued for the relief it brings from Inner Critic inflicted emotional pain. The result is that each type becomes a characterological state relied upon for daily functioning.

In addition, the Inner Critic functions by imposing Cherished Dysfunctional Beliefs, which consist of shoulds and shouldn'ts that create the polar types. What makes the beliefs cherished is the fact that the person finds them valuable as a support for self-esteem. In order to create an HVR, each partner must shift to holding such cherished beliefs in a provisional manner.

Avoiding Universal Prescriptions

Clinical experience indicates that there is no universal prescription for any one person's growth. As they obey the commands of the Inner Critic, each of the four polar types has submerged the energies that are the polar opposite of what is hyper-cultivated. Therefore, each type submerges different energies. The task of growth toward optimal functioning is to reclaim whatever energies have been idiosyncratically submerged and disowned.

Creation of Lacunae

As long as the person's energies are submerged, the person's Inner Critic will drive him or her to compulsively maintain the submergence. This drivenness will exhibit itself in therapy in the form of lucanae, which are gaps in the person's repertoire of thoughts, feelings, attitudes, and behaviors.

The Tough type will be unable to be Tender. The Tender type will have difficulty being Tough. The Dependent Type will have problems with independent thought and action. The Self-Sufficient type will have difficulties with closeness.

The low-voltage person is apt to be Self-Sufficient. The LV individual will possess little access to Dependent neediness.

The creation of lacunae in the self-structure will occur through fear. That is, if a gap occurs, it will be because the person feels anxiety induced by the threat of Inner Critic emotional punishment were the gap to be filled.

Each fear is a clue to the kind of polar type the person has adopted. For example, the Tough type is afraid of losing control. The Tender type is afraid of being insensitive and unloving. The Dependent type is afraid of losing approval and emotional support. The Self-Sufficient type is afraid of losing independence.

However, each polar type personality may not be in touch with those fears. This is because the polar type behavior is a defense against ever experiencing the fear and having to cope with the pain.

Facilitating Repertoire Expansion

As the therapist helps partners become free of their hyper-cultivated polar rigidities, it is important to note that no polar style is terminal. Each rigidity was learned, and each can be unlearned. The goal of growth, then, is to unlearn the rigid styles adopted in order to maximize options for deploying the four types.

In other words, the goal here is *psychological flexibility*. Note that the goal is not balance, not finding a midpoint in a continuum and consistently choosing a happy medium. Instead, the goal is disengaging from the entire continuum so that, from an orthogonal (i.e., perpendicular or right-angle) position, the partner can choose any point he or she wishes on the continuum.

Implications for optimal relating are that in order to have an HVR, partners must be able to access and deploy any one of the four polar styles whenever they choose. Optimally, once free from Inner Critic induce polar rigidity, partners may be able to choose assertiveness (Tough), melting love and empathy (Tender), neediness and longing (Dependence), and comfortableness in being alone (Self-Sufficient).

In order to facilitate such flexibility, the therapist must also gain freedom from polar rigidity developed in his or her life.

THE PURSUER-DISTANCER PATTERN

At the heart of a well-known malady in romantic relationships is the Pursuer-Distancer pattern, also termed the Demand-Withdraw pattern. In such dyadic relationships one person tends to pursue, while the other tends to withdraw (Berns, Jacobson, & Gottman, 1999; Christensen & Heavey, 1993). In extreme cases the Distancer says, "She wants too much; I feel suffocated." The Pursuer says, "I want so little, and I don't even get *that.*" Explanations for this pattern have centered on the impact of social norms and gender-based differences in that many wives exhibit the Demand or Pursuer role, while their husbands respond with the Withdraw or Distancer role. A structural explanation challenges this social normative perspective and posits that the interdependent nature of marriage is based on the allocation of resources to meet partners' wants and needs, and that the demand-withdraw pattern is fueled more by interdependence structure in close relationships than by social norms or personal dispositions (Rusbult, Kumashiro, Coolsen, & Kirchner, 2004).

The Anthetic Relationship typology of the Four Polar Types offers a psychodynamic understanding for the subconscious structure driving both the Pursuer and Distancer. Applying the template of the polar types, the Pursuer can be seen as a Dependent type; the Distancer is Self-Sufficient. The more intense the pursuit, the more anxiety the Distancer feels with a resulting further distancing. The process escalates. The Self-Sufficient partner does not see the Dependent person's actions as loving or desperate moves toward closeness, that is, as a wish for high voltage. Instead, the Self-Sufficient interprets overtures for closeness as intrusive, demanding, and controlling and responds by retreating further. The Self-Sufficient person comes to three conclusions: First, "No, matter how much I give, she'll always want more"; second, "I'll never be able to meet her demands, so why try"; and third, "I'll give up and retreat behind my walls."

The role of the therapist with a couple who have entered a therapeutic contract for more closeness is to offer the Self-Sufficient partner concepts and skills for understanding and becoming free from the rigid defensive structure from which he or she operates. Central to the Anthetic Therapy conceptualization of the Self-Sufficient partner's distancing is the understanding that he or she simply lacks skills for being close and still free. The psychological structure underlying this dynamic centers in the Inner Critic, which has imposed shoulds to be Tender, self-effacing, and non-assertive. Contrary to a Tender person who received reinforcement for being tender, the Self-Sufficient was hurt when tender. This emotional pain became too great to continue in the Tender pattern resulting in the defensive solution of distancing. This Self-Sufficient structure calcified into a rigid solution relied upon when the stress of intimate relating became too anxiety-provoking.

A complicating factor in the Distancer's response is often the Tender Dependent pursuer's judgmentalism ("Come on, stop clamming up; open up!"). Exposed to such judgmentalism, the Self-Sufficient partner feels raw. The therapist must equip the Self-Sufficient with the Anthetic releasing statements that can help him maintain his or her equanimity. At the same time, the therapist teaches the Pursuer to become free from Inner Critic commands underlying the judgmentalism. Whereas Johnson's (2004) *Emotionally Focused Therapy for Couples* addresses the Pursuer-Distancer pattern through a method of therapist *softening* partners toward each other utilizing a strategy of empathy and reframing, the Anthetic Relationship Therapy approach offers the couple *skills* for dismantling the driving psychodynamic structure of the P-D pattern.

The Pursuer-Distancer pattern becomes understandable when seen from the perspective of Anthetic voltage theory. The Inner Critic is the ultimate source of this dyadic style. It is the Inner Critic commanding the Distancer to withdraw. As the therapist guides the Distancing partner in Anthetic Dialogue to voice idiosyncratic shoulds, specific releasing statements can be formulated for becoming free from the driving power of the shoulds. In addition to gaining such intrapsychic skills, the Distancer also learns interpersonal skills (to be covered in Chapters 8 and 9) for enjoying closeness while retaining freedom.

The crucial role of Anthetic Inner Critic work becomes evident as partners' counter-humiliation strategies become dismantled, empowering them to access all four polarities and deploy previously submerged elements as needed in the relationship.

Chapter 4

Using the Anthetic Inner Figure Language

Across the span of the development of approaches for working with intrapsychic processes, a revolution emerged in the field of psychotherapy: the transition from a "monoself" language to what can be called a "multifigure" language. Initially, mainstream psychotherapy had understood the person as a single entity. When a person feels angry, he or she is the one who is angry. When one feels hurt, it is a single "you" who feels hurt. When one feels anxious, it is the total person who feels anxious. That is, these feelings are "states of mind."

In other words, an individual is seen as a single personality who has first one feeling, then another, then still another, and so on, each feeling replacing the previous one. The model is a linear one. Anthetic Psychology views the self not as a single entity but as a mosaic—a collection of simultaneously occurring elements called inner figures. In order to achieve an HVR, the person must become proficient in speaking this inner figure language. This conceptualization is essential to the feedback process in which partners engage in psychological growth. In clinical experience, most partners' blocks to living out the value of optimality and high-voltage relating can be removed using inner figure work with the couple.

These inner figures are parts of the person; referred to by partners even prior to learning the language when they say, "Part of me wants to move to a large city; part of me wants to live in the country." In other words, people talk about inner figures all the time without always knowing it.

INNER FIGURES IN PSYCHOTHERAPY

Psychotherapies that use the vocabulary of self-parts have offered varying terms to describe them. What Anthetic Therapy calls inner figures have been referred to by Freud (1923/1949) as agencies and by post-Freudian theorists, including Melanie Klein as "objects", introjected representations of significant people in a person's life (Klein, 1948; Gunthrip, 1971). Jung (1935/1968) wrote of the infinite number of complexes and archetypes each person has, which he viewed as more than introjects, but rather "fragmentary" or "partial" personalities (pp. 80–81). Robert Assagioli (1965) referred to a collection of subpersonalities. Eric Berne (1961, 1972) offered ego states; Fritz Perls (1969) wrote about the top dog and underdog. Cognitive-behavioral therapists describe possible selves (Markus & Nurius, 1987). Primary within the field of family therapy is the Internal Family Systems model of Richard Schwartz (1995), the emphasis of which is the network of relationships of parts. Each part comprises "a discrete and autonomous mental system that has an idiosyncratic range of emotion, style of expression, set of abilities, desires, and views of the world" (p. 34). Also emerging in understanding the mind from the standpoint of multiplicity is research on the brain. One such researcher, Gazzaniga (1985), poses that the mind consists of modules, which he describes as independently functioning units that each plays a special role. Similar to Schwartz, Gazzaniga holds that emotion and cognition are shaped by the relationship among the modules.

Unique in the field of multiself models, Anthetic Psychology holds that the Inner Critic is a key inner figure in understanding personality dynamics (Chapter 3). The present chapter will describe more inner figures and their role in the HVR.

What is An Inner Figure?

Each inner figure is a complex configuration of related elements, among which are feelings, concepts, thoughts, beliefs, impulses, desires, behavior patterns, attitudes, decisions, archetypes, attachments, somatic elements, images, fantasies, and symbols.

The inner figure is semi-autonomous; that is, it seems to have a mind of its own and purposes of its own. At the same time, it can be influenced by its "owner." It can also be submerged in the subconscious part of the psyche, resulting in the individual being unaware of it. Once given feedback about it, however, the inner figure can become conscious.

For any inner figure, the related elements seem to "go together," in the sense that they appear meaningfully connected. For example, in an Angry

Child there will be angry feelings, angry behavior, tightening of body muscles, an impulse to hit, and a memory of parental anger as a model. Any figure may or may not be expressed in behavior; that is, it may simply exist as a part that never gets to play a role in the person's life. One word about the ontological status of inner figures seems fitting here. Anthetic Therapy holds that inner figures exist not in the physicalist domain but in the mentalist domain of subjective reality.

An additional issue often asked by clients when introduced to the concept of inner figures is, "Do inner figures exist in normal people or do I have multiple personality disorder?" Anthetic Therapy, along with most multiplicity of self models, holds that "normal" people have inner figures, as their personalities consist of parts. However, in most people inner figures are submerged in the subconscious levels of the psyche. From this deeper level, they influence the thoughts, feelings, behaviors, and attitudes of the person, usually without that person's awareness of what is happening. In contrast to individuals with Dissociative Identity Disorder, those without the disorder have a primary organizing figure, the Executive Self who is aware of or can become aware of the person's behavior and can direct any figure's actions.

The process is one of fusion; that is, people can be fused with their inner figures. The more of these fusions that exist, the more difficult it will be for the person to think clearly. Instead, they will be pushed around by their impulses. The result is reactivity. Clients report that use of the inner figure language in their own therapeutic process results in greater clarity as well as an ability to sort out their thoughts and feelings. The ultimate benefit they report is a greater ability to make decisions, clear of confusion.

Who "Has" the Inner Figures?

Who "owns" the inner figures? An examination of the ontological status of that which is the "I" in "I own it" seems to be in order here. Clearly, it cannot be another inner figure, because then there would arise the question, "Well, so who owns that one?" The question could then be asked repeatedly resulting in an infinite regress.

What is needed is a theory that can be tested by pragmatic methods: What works best in actual practice? In other words, what makes sense of all these figures? Anthetic Psychology proposes the following principle: That which "has" the inner figures must be that which transcends all the figures and is never one of them. Anthetic Psychology refers to it as the Transcendental Self, or T-self (Elliott, J., & Elliott, K., 2000). It is who the individual is apart from his or her inner figures, a core self. This T-self can never actually be perceived by the individual because it is the self who does the perceiving of the inner figures.

Principles are needed to convert this process into a practical one:

1. The individual, as the T-self, has the ability to fuse with any inner figure. In addition, the individual has the ability to disengage from it, using the Anthetic Dialogue method (Elliott, J., 1992b)
2. Having fused with an inner figure, the individual thinks he or she *is* the inner figure. For example, if one is resistant to processing feedback, such resistance is a clue that the person has become fused with an inner Resistant Child.
3. Each fusion results in a loss of a portion of one's inner freedom. That is, in rigidity in the individual. He or she will now be driven by the inner figure with which fused. In the example above, the fusion may make it difficult or impossible to overcome resistance to learning to do the processing.
4. This perspective holds that resistance is a state of mind, not an element in one's mind. It pervades one's entire consciousness. The person does not see the resistance as a problem; it is ego-syntonic. What the individual sees instead is the other person to whom he or she is resistant. In the field of the individual's perception, the other is seen as a "bad" person; someone who is trying to put something over one. The feedback is then seen as an accusation, or a punishment, not a course correction.
5. However, when the individual engages in Anthetic Dialogue and carries on a conversation with the Resistant Child, the status of the inner figure changes from a state of mind to an element in the mind. As an element, the figure is easier to work with in psychotherapy.
6. Through Anthetic Dialoguing, the person has begun to disengage from the resistant inner figure. Rigidity reduces, and inner freedom from the element increases.
7. This procedure can be applied to anything with which one is fused (i.e., attached): pride, anger, infatuation, self-centeredness, guilt feelings, or the Inner Critic. Disengaging is a powerful new method for achieving inner freedom.
8. This theory permits a view of growth as consisting of a series of unlayerings or exfoliations. With each exfoliation of that to which one was attached, the person becomes more and more free.

   Will the person ever reach the T-self? The answer is probably not. However, as the person becomes asymptotically closer to the goal of disengagement, he or she reduces blocks to optimal functioning. The person becomes less reactive, less like a jukebox whose buttons anyone may push.
9. From the position of disengagement from the inner figures, the individual is now free to merge with any one of them. From the position of the T-self, free choice occurs in which the individual may choose to actualize that from which one is disengaged, whether resistance, anger, love, or

assertiveness. Now the merging occurs through free choice rather than as a driven, reactive process outside the person's conscious control.

10. Some inner figures are negative, some are positive. Anthetic therapy recommends one not try to change or transform negative inner figures, instead to replace such figures with a different figure. For example, if a person has isolated an inner figure that procrastinates, rather than making it more responsible and effective, replace it with a responsible and effective inner figure. In this way, all the figures retain their original format. Clinical experience indicates that inner figures do not change, but rather become submerged in their original form, operating outside of awareness.

Still, a reactive inner figure can be drained of its energy. The figure will still be there, but will be unable to impact one's life.

Four Categories of Inner Figures

Anthetic Psychology classifies inner figures in four categories: inner figures in the Natural Self (positive inner figures); the Rational Self; the Inner Critic (a negative inner figure); and reactive inner figures generated in response to the Inner Critic (negative inner figures manifested in dysfunctionality).

The Natural Self (sometimes referred to as "the authentic self") contains all the vital energies the individual had as a child, before the Inner Critic developed and exerted its influence. It is rich with possibilities for a happy and satisfying life. The Natural Self is made up of the primary self and secondary self, containing all the vital energies of the primary self plus the structure of the secondary self used to deploy those energies (Elliott, J., & Elliott, K., 2000). The Anthetic concept of the primary self is much like the Freudian concept of primary process. The latter is a mode of functioning of the psyche characterized by an urgency for tension reduction without regard for external reality (Freud (1900/1955, p. 601; 1915/1957, pp. 186f). The Anthetic concept of the primary self is somewhat like the Transactional Analysis concept of the Natural Child (Berne, 1961). Secondary self structure is akin to the Freudian concept of secondary process, characterized by delay of gratification of needs and wishes (Freud 1915/1957, pp. 186f; 1900/1955, p. 601). Its function is to channel and focus primary self energies to match them to the environment, thereby satisfying the primary needs. The secondary self is somewhat like the Transactional Analysis concept of script, provided one distinguishes between what might be called a driven script and a free script. Anthetics holds that the secondary self is partly free, partly driven (Elliott, J., & Elliott, K., 2000). Among the inner figures included in the Natural Self are the Playful Child, the Loving Child, the Sexual Self, and the Creative Self. The Natural Self wants pleasure and satisfaction.

The Rational Self, sometimes called the Realistic Self, is concerned with accurately processing information, solving problems, anticipating consequences of possible decisions, clearing misconceptions and other dysfunctional thoughts, and constructing and testing hypotheses and theories not only about scientific topics but also about everyday life. The term *task oriented* may also be used to describe the Rational Self, because its goal is to stay on task and not be diverted by illusions, logical fallacies, wishful thinking, defensiveness, pulls to defend and protect the self-image, and other forms of reactivity. The Rational Self is not synonymous with the Adult of Transactional Analysis, which translates rationality with the developmental stage of being grownup. In Anthetic theory, the Rational Self is merely the Rational part of the individual: neither Parent, Adult, nor Child.

The Inner Critic (discussed more fully in Chapter 3) is an Anthetic archetype. Anthetic Therapy derives its archetypes from the Anthetic Dialogue process, rather than from accounts of dreams, religions, and myths. What Jung called the archetype is known in Anthetic Therapy as the archetypal matrix. In contrast to Jung's commitment to Kantian dualism which caused him to see the archetype as a noumenon which was represented in experience by symbols and images, Anthetic Therapy holds that the archetype *is* the inner figure that appears in Anthetic Dialogue.

Emotional seepage is said to happen when strong reactive emotions seep from the sub-system of the Reactive Emotional Self into the Rational Self. In order for the person to think clearly, these emotions must be identified and their saliency reduced. A corollary of this position is the recommendation that one not debate or argue with a partner whose emotions are running high, because such a person will not be able to do task-oriented processing of what is said. Being task-oriented does not mean insulating oneself from the feelings and impulses of the Natural Self. It means taking these feelings into account and evaluating them rationally. (See Chapter 6, "Using the Anthetic Rationality Sequence.")

INNER FIGURES AND THE HIGH-VOLTAGE RELATIONSHIP

Inner figures are an essential element in creating the HVR for several reasons. First, they play an important role in partner choice. For the single person aware of his or her voltage preference, it is best if the Natural Self, guided by the Rational Self, seeks a partner who shares a preference for high voltage. The therapist can assist the individual in evaluating potential partners by helping articulate criteria for a partner (Elliott, J., & Elliott, K., 2010). In addition, the therapist can empower the individual to identify reactive inner figures, such as an Infatuated Child, who through its longing for love along with its unwillingness to consult with the Rational Self, influences the person to pick a partner based merely on impulse or chemistry. Second, once a person is in a relationship, inner figures feature prominently in achieving high-voltage relating. For example, when an argument has ensued, an inner figure such as a Vengeful Child can lead a partner to reject overtures for reconciliation and resolution of the conflict. As this occurs repetitively, partners no longer create a safe haven for closeness, but rather an adversarial climate leading to distance and low-voltage.

Advantages of the Multifigure Language

The multifigure language is simply one language among many for thinking and talking about psychological matters. By contrast, "feeling language" uses a different vocabulary to talk about the same things. For example, if one wants to understand why someone seeks revenge, feeling terms can be used to say, "Because he feels angry and wants justice." For complex cases involving more than one feeling, psychotherapists often use feeling language plus the concept of ambivalence: "My client wants to get married, but she's afraid to make a commitment, and in addition, she feels guilty about leaving her parents. She's ambivalent." Such a statement of ambivalence can be translated from feeling language into inner figure language as follows: "Part of the client wants to get married; part of her fears commitment; and part of her feels guilty." Each part, of course, is an inner figure.

Inner figure language has a number of advantages in clinical utility over the language of feelings only. First, inner figure language offers items that have dynamic interconnections among phenomena that might initially appear to be unconnected. For example, if part of a person fears intimacy, that part can be seen in terms of a pattern that will probably include more than feelings. It will have aspects having to do with thoughts, perceptions, somatic elements (e.g., sensations and body armoring), fantasies, images, memories, predictions, and early decisions. It will also have its own particular cherished dysfunctional beliefs. If these are all seen as elements of an inner figure, the therapist can assist the person to search for and uncover each element and then understand how they interact.

A second advantage of inner figure language is that it often is familiar to clients in therapy. For example, the client may have thought, "Part of me wants to stay home and study; part of me wants to go to the party." The therapist can point out that such parlance is inner figure language.

A third advantage is that inner figure work neatly undercuts the "what's *really* going on" issue common in couple therapy. For example, if one partner feels anger, the other partner may say, "What you are *really* feeling is hurt."

Hearing this, the angry partner may disown the "non-real" feeling and miss the opportunity to gain insight and freedom from anger as well as hurt.

Inner figure theory permits therapist and client to think in terms of having several parts, perhaps one of which feels anger, while another feels hurt. Thus there is no longer an issue of which is real; they both are. Using feeling language only, the client may be confused about how to think about multiple feelings (e.g., "How can I feel both love and anger for the same person?").

Closely related to this issue is a fourth advantage of inner figure language. When partners learn the inner figure language in couple therapy, it helps them reframe and defuse a common source of conflict. The conflict occurs when one partner makes a request of the other, who agrees to the request, whereupon the requesting partner says, "Well, you said you'd do it, all right, but you don't *really* want to do it." Inner figure language permits the requestee to then say, "Sure. Part of me does, part of me doesn't, but I agreed to do it, and I will. It's not a question of 'really' or 'not really' wanting to."

A fifth advantage of inner figure language is that it lends itself well to giving effective feedback. For example, saying "You're in your Little Girl" indicates the constellation that is usually immediately apparent to both partners. This constellation might include anxiety, fuzzy thinking, anger, hurt feelings, and replay elements.

A sixth advantage of this language, and perhaps the most important one, is that if the client and therapist think in terms of inner figures, they can use Anthetic Dialogue to work with each inner figure imagined as occupying an empty chair. It tends to be more productive clinically to dialogue with an inner figure rather than with a feeling.

A seventh advantage is that once Inner Figure dialogue takes place, a process called Inner Figure Orchestration (to be described later) can be done. In Anthetic Therapy, Inner Figure Orchestration is the method of choice for overcoming difficult problems.

An eighth advantage is based on the fact that psychotherapy of any kind tends to trigger fear as well as to elicit emotional pain. Anthetic Inner Critic Work helps reduce or eliminate this pain, since it is the Inner Critic that causes the pain. Doing therapy without directly addressing this inner figure is like doing surgery without an anesthetic.

To overcome the effects of dysfunctionality, each inner figure must be addressed using a different strategy. For example, if a person is hurt and angry, the method to be used with the hurt inner figure will differ from the method for the angry inner figure.

A ninth advantage is that if the therapist and client use inner figure language, the client can be helped to identify the "pull" of a dysfunctional inner figure and resist that pull. For example, Claudette's husband, Kevin, asked her what she thought of a report he had written for his boss. She felt a temptation (a pull) to be dishonest and say the report was great. The pull was exerted by her obedient Little Girl who was responding to a should to avoid upsetting Kevin. She decided to resist the pull and tell the truth: the report was seriously disorganized. She expected that Kevin would be touchy and angry upon receiving this feedback, but instead he was grateful. In other words, she thought he would be someone with whom she had to tread carefully. However, it was merely her Inner Critic's prediction of catastrophe. She then began a program of taking more risks in truth-telling, and although some of her attempts triggered Kevin's anger, she was able to tell him, "I think you're in your Little Boy right now." Kevin in turn appreciated the feedback, because both he and Claudette had been learning feedback processing skills (Chapter 5) and were in agreement on the values needed to support those skills.

Finally, a tenth advantage is that if therapy involves the use of inner figure vocabulary, clients can benefit from a method called Re-attribution Processing to work with the pain of receiving certain kinds of feedback. Re-attribution Processing means shifting the perceived location of the cause of pain from "the person who gave me the feedback" to "my Inner Critic." This will enable the therapist and client to focus the therapeutic work on the correct cause of distress: the client's Inner Critic.

Inner Figure Orchestration

Inner Figure Orchestration is a strategy in which the person first recognizes or perceives the inner figure clearly. Second, the therapist helps the client isolate the figure: naming it, describing its features, liberating the energy bound in it, understanding the relationships among its elements, assessing the positive and negative consequences of deploying it, and seeing the relationships between the inner figure and other inner figures. Then third, the therapist assists the person to orchestrate it; that is, decide whether and how to deploy the inner figure's energies in constructive ways. This three part process once learned in therapy is portable. The client and the couple can utilize it in their everyday lives apart from therapy.

As orchestration proceeds, some of the inner figures can be assigned various roles in the client's life or no roles at all. For example, if the client reports feeling disempowered in relationships, the therapist can help the client access the Disempowered Self, analyze it, and direct it to remain out of play in behavior. The same process can be done with the Angry Child and the Judgmental Child. At the same time, the client may access the Powerful Self or Loving Self and give them prominent roles in his or her life.

In Inner Figure Orchestration, the client dialogues with the inner figure, telling it what part to play in his or her life, if any. The process is not one of asking permission but rather of directing or commanding it. Moreover, the inner figure is never eliminated. The person merely has a new relationship with it, taking charge of it rather than the figure taking charge of the person.

Identifying an Inner Figure

As mentioned earlier, entities in one's inner world do not exhibit the same kind of reality as entities in the outer material world. There is an ontological difference: the inner figure has subjective reality.

In the material world, entities are relatively stable. In the inner world, they are amorphous. What counts as an entity seems to depend, to a large extent, on how one thinks about it. That is, a person can actually change an inner figure simply by a thought process. One can, for example, speak as though there is only one Inner Child figure, having aspects (e.go., being self-effacing, feeling hurt, feeling angry). Alternatively, one can construe this entity as divided into three Inner Child figures; one who is self-effacing, one who is hurt, and one who is angry. Anthetic Therapy finds greater clinical utility in dialoguing with a "pure" or discrete inner figure, for example, an Angry Child.

Reactive Inner Figures

As mentioned in Chapter 3, the Inner Critic's goal is to sabotage relationships by enforcing injunctions that are designed to constrict one's options. Typically, the person will not be aware of the Inner Critic as the source of these injunctions. Nor will he or she be aware of the dysfunctional consequences of buying into the injunctions. They will seem perfectly normal and even in some cases helpful.

The person may become aware of these processes when the Anthetic therapist uses special methods to help identify the injunctions, whereupon he or she can become free from them. Until that point, the Inner Critic will proceed to create reactive inner figures that constitute additional emotional obstacles to achieving the HVR. Clinical experience indicates that most partners exhibit relating from the reactive figures of the Dysfunctional Little Boy or Girl. Each of these figures is the source of reactivity that becomes acted out in the relationship, whether judgmentalism, anger, vindictiveness, or disempowerment. Other frequently occurring reactive figures include negative introjects from childhood (Mom, Dad, or other powerful relatives or teachers), other negative personal figures from the present or recent past (a tyrannical boss, a former therapist who was judgmental), negative spiritual figures (a punitive God, Satan), or reactive personae (e.g., "The Doormat," "The Moralist").

A Case Example of Inner Figures in Couple Therapy

Gabi and Ted, married 27 years, sought couple counseling for repetitive escalating arguments. Ted was first to speak, "We have differences of opinion that escalate into an argument. She feels strongly one way, and I feel another." Gabi quickly followed with, "He interrupts. He likes to fight. He likes me to be upset. I simply offer a suggestion, and he immediately starts shaking his head and says, 'You're trying to push that on me.' I can't freely be who I want to be. Then, he's so worried about money that I can't suggest we buy anything for our new house. I'm stressed out. It's making me sick." Ted responded, "I'm the breadwinner, and I get so worried about money. She does try to be careful about costs, but she's always finding something else we need." Both asserted that they loved each other and though significantly stressed by their conflict, wanted to stay together and work things out.

Anthetic Dialogue revealed salient Inner Figures functioning in both partners.

The therapist first moved Gabi to an orthogonal position to observe the part who had been speaking.

Therapist: Gabi, as you look at the person who was sitting there talking, can you see her?

Gabi: Oh, yes! (with a wry laugh)

Therapist: Let's talk about her characteristics. How would you describe her?

Gabi: Well, she seems to feel less power than Ted. And she's tired. She walks on eggshells, always trying to avoid saying something that will set him off.

Therapist: Yes, and she said, "He likes to fight. He likes me to be upset."

Gabi: Yes.

(At this point, the therapist perceives an opening to explore the psychodynamic roots of this inner figure.)

Therapist: Is this a new or an old feeling that she is feeling?

Gabi: I'd say it is old. We've been married 27 years, and it's been this way since the beginning.

Therapist: And as you look at her, was the beginning of her marriage the first time you had felt that way or can you remember an even earlier time when you had the feelings she has?

Gabi: Well, when I was growing up, my father drank. He would get drunk and chase my mother with a broom, beating her with it. I watched all this. I'd try to protect my mother. (crying) I'd plead with him, 'Dad, don't do that!' But he didn't care that I was upset. He'd just keep chasing Mom.

Therapist: So, when you look at this figure who says, 'He likes to fight; he likes me to be upset,' does it look and feel like the same feelings when Dad ignored your pleas; seeming not to care what you felt?

Gabi: Why, yes, it feels very much like that. My gosh, I had never realized that!

Therapist: Is it a surprising connection for you?

Gabi: Yes, it is! And a helpful one.

Therapist: How old would you say this part of you is?

Gabi: Well, in the memory I have of Dad chasing Mom down the driveway (and it's a vivid one), I'm about 15.

Therapist: So, can you see that this is the 15 year old part of you who felt so powerless to get Dad to attend to her distress?

Gabi: Yes.

Therapist: She is a part of you; an inner figure, who has these memories, feelings, perspectives. What can you call her?

Gabi: I think I'll just call her Dad's Daughter.

(The perspective-taking of the orthogonal technique has now allowed Gabi to see and name this part of her. The therapist now mobilizes Gabi's empathic and executive functions in order to move to orchestrating the inner figure.)

Therapist: What feelings are you having toward Dad's Daughter?

Gabi: I feel for her (tears).

Therapist: Would you tell her, 'I feel for you;' 'I'm so sorry you went through that'?

Gabi: I do. I feel for you. I *am* sorry you went through that. It was painful for you that you couldn't protect your mom. And you couldn't get your dad to hear you.

(At this point, the therapist facilitates an orchestration of the inner figure in regard to Gabi's relationship with her husband.)

Therapist: Would you tell Dad's Daughter whether she needs to be the one to handle the discussions you have with Ted?

Gabi: (Surprised; puzzled) Whether *she* needs to be the one to have discussions with Ted?

Therapist: (Clarifying) Yes, is the 15 year old Dad's Daughter equipped to handle the discussions and negotiations of a husband and wife?

Gabi: (Realization dawning) Oh! (Chuckling) Oh, no, Dad's Daughter, you don't need to handle these discussions at all!

Therapist: Yes, tell her whether another part of you who has more life experience, insight, skill, and wisdom will handle those.

Gabi: Yes! I'll handle those from the skills and wisdom I'm learning in therapy and from all the years of learning I've had.

Therapist: Yes, and I will be teaching you these skills.

Therapist: When Dad's Daughter gets triggered, is there a characteristic feeling or thought you have that can help you know when she is coming on stage?

Gabi: Oh, yes. I felt tense; heaviness in my chest; like it's hard to breathe.

Therapist: So, when you and Ted begin to have a discussion about a purchase or other issue, you can now be watching for those characteristic feelings. Then you can do two things: First, label the feelings. Oh, this is Dad's Daughter coming on stage. Second, in order to not fuse with her, you can get up and move, then look back at where Dad's Daughter is and tell her, 'You don't need to handle this.'

Gabi: (laughing) Yes, I can tell her, 'You can go and read a fashion magazine or polish your nails!'

Therapist: Exactly! Then you can call on the part of you who is learning skills in couple therapy and have her be the one discussing with Ted.

Gabi: Sounds great! I like this!

Therapist (to Ted): You mentioned that you feel worried about money when Gabi brings up a house purchase.

Ted: I do. I just feel afraid we won't have enough money to pay the bills. It's all up to me.

Therapist (directing Ted in Anthetic Dialogue): Ted, would you sit here now? (Pointing to a chair in an orthogonal position to which Ted moves)

Therapist: Can you describe the person who was sitting here?

Ted: He's a mess! He gets so worried. And then it starts a big fight with Gabi.

Therapist: Gabi said that you immediately start shaking your head. Can you do that now?

Ted shakes his head back and forth; his chin down.

Therapist: What words would you like to say as you shake your head?

Ted: I get to have an opinion too, don't I?

Therapist: Ted, does this feeling of worry over money and protesting that you get to have an opinion feel new or old?

Ted: Oh, it feels old.

Gabi (to Ted): Tell her about your childhood.

Ted: Well, my dad died when I was 10 years old. I was the oldest of five kids, and it fell to me to be sort of the man of the house. I had to take jobs after school. Mom would tell me all her worries about money.

Therapist: Does it fit that the feelings you had at 10 are the feelings you have when you and Gabi start to discuss purchases?

Ted: (Surprised) Why, yes it does! I even start feeling that pit in my stomach when Gabi brings up buying something.

Therapist: So, the part of you who gets triggered by conversations that involve money is the 10 year old son.

Ted: Yes, it seems so.

Therapist: Can you give him a name?

Ted: Yes, I'll just call him 'My Kid.'

Therapist: Do you feel some empathy for My Kid; for the boy who lived through that?

Ted: Yes, I do.

Therapist: Would you tell him, 'I'm so sorry you went through that,' or whatever feels right to you?

Ted: I *am* sorry you went through that. You were pushed to give up your childhood and become Mom's help; her sounding board.

Therapist: Do you want My Kid to be the one who handles your discussions with Gabi about money and purchases?

Ted: No, My Kid, you don't need to handle those conversations. You had enough of that. You need to just enjoy your childhood.

Therapist: Ted, I want to give you the two step process to do when you feel My Kid coming on stage. When you feel that pit in your stomach, first label it, "That's My Kid." Then, second, tell My Kid, "You can go out and play. I'll handle this discussion from the adult part of me who is learning skills in therapy."

Ted: Ok, I can do that. That's pretty neat.

Therapist: So, Gabi and Ted, can you see that the people who have been living your marriage, at least in the area of money, were two inner figures from your childhoods?

Gabi and Ted: Yes! That is amazing!

Therapist: Now, you can use the two part inner figure protocol to make space for a skillful conversation. Simply, suspend content, and disengage from the inner figures of Dad's Daughter and My Kid. If you would like to begin doing this at home, would you turn and tell each other. (They do so.)

Gabi (to Ted): I want to get Dad's Daughter off-stage so we can have productive discussions that stay loving.

Ted (to Gabi): Me too. I want to get out of My Kid so we can relate from our adults and not end up in a fight.

As the session ends, the therapist encourages the couple that repetition of catching the inner figures and orchestrating them will help them stay out of conflict and remain task oriented and loving.

As the case of Gabi and Ted illustrates, intrapsychic work entailed in Inner Figure identification and orchestration can be the turning point in couple therapy. The disengagement from reactive self structure in each partner enables access to rational and loving communication.

Part II

CREATING THE HIGH-VOLTAGE RELATIONSHIP

Chapter 5

What It Takes to Create a High-Voltage Relationship

The Anthetic Values

Clinical experience has shown that a desire for or attraction to an HVR, while an important first step, is insufficient for actually creating one. Couples who declare an interest in doing so cannot actualize their desire through a simple decision to do so. The initial step involves adopting new values, that is, accepting being guided by values that support a growth-centered relationship. Once a couple accepts these values, they can use them as guides to their behavior. In addition, the therapist can use the couple's acceptance of the values as a guide to the principles and skills to teach the couple. Moreover, at those times when the couple becomes troubled by reactive or destructive patterns, either the partners or the therapist may invoke the values to further the process of movement toward high-voltage relating.

The sequence for creating an HVR involves three steps. First, partners accept the basic guidelines (concepts, values, and principles). Second, both partners learn the skills for psychological work on oneself (intrapersonal skills). Third, the couple learns the high-voltage communication skills (interpersonal skills).

An important guiding factor in choosing high-voltage values is differential source of motivation. Clinical experience indicates that optimal relating, and specifically high-voltage relating, requires greater than normal desire for closeness, along with an enthusiastic commitment to the values. In addition, partners' desire for an HVR must come from their Natural Selves, guided by their Executive Selves, not from shoulds of their Reactive Selves. An important indicator that motivation is coming from partners' Natural Selves is that they will report pleasure in taking the steps necessary to achieve the HVR. If, on the other hand, the couple adopts the values only from shoulds, or to look good, or to get credit from their partners or the therapist, the values and skills will eventually feel like burdensome chores. Successful HVRs are characterized by partners' reporting feeling excited, self-motivated, and personally owning the process whether they receive credit, support, or encouragement for doing so.

Value 1: Inner Freedom

Foundational to creating an HVR is holding the value of Inner Freedom. Inner Freedom includes freedom from hyper-attachments of all kinds, but most important, freedom from attachment to the Inner Critic. Hyper-attachment is synonymous with fusion. Opposite to hyper-attachment are disengagement, separation, and differentiation. Note that inner freedom is not synonymous with detachment, which is a more radical and sometimes crystallized form of separation.

Valuing inner freedom as well as learning the skills for achieving it are necessary for the couple not only to tolerate but also to actually enjoy the intensity of high-voltage relating, for example, receiving disconfirmatory feedback. Without valuing inner freedom, partners become defensive when given feedback. In addition, without this value, the couple will seek a cosmetic therapy approach as a method of personal change, merely shaping and constricting themselves in a futile attempt to achieve closeness. Once owning the value of inner freedom, partners seek a transformative therapy approach in which psychological symptoms are seen as clues to deeper functioning or dysfunctioning.

Value 2: Safe Haven vs. Combat Relationship

In coping with conflict, low-voltage partners usually rely on one of three options: fighting, submitting, or distancing. Distancing becomes a coping strategy to avoid either fighting or submitting.

In order to create high-voltage, on the other hand, couples share the value of creating their relationship as a safe haven, in which they feel safe enough to talk about anything, especially feelings. A safe haven is one in which partners may enjoy emotional closeness, soft-heartedness, and love. A combat relationship is one in which verbal attacking via anger, judgmentalism, and blaming has become accepted as normal.

Value 3: Emotional Closeness

While research on closeness reveals that no single common conceptualization exists within the fields that study relationships nor among those fields, certain common themes do appear in the vast volume of research on closeness and intimacy (Aron & Mashek, 2004). These themes include interdependency, mutual influence, and cognitive connectedness of selves (Agnew, Loving, Le, & Goodfriend, 2004; Arriaga, Goodfriend, & Lohmann, 2004; Aron, Mashek, & Aron, 2004; Berscheid, Snyder & Omoto, 2004; Ickes, Hutchison, & Mashek, 2004; Mashek & Sherman, 2004; Rusbult, Kumashiro, Coolsen, & Kirchner, 2004). Other researchers emphasize intimacy based on self-disclosure, responsiveness, vulnerabilities, mutual understanding, touching, social support, and caring (Fehr, 2004; Firestone, R.W., & Firestone, L., 2004; Kouneski & Olson, 2004; Prager & Roberts, 2004; Laurenceau, Rivera, Schaffer, & Pietromonaco, 2004; Reis, Clark, & Holmes, 2004; Sanderson, 2004; Vohs & Baumeister, 2004).

Anthetic Relationship Therapy agrees with the previous researchers and holds that closeness is characterized by the following elements: openness, quotidian honesty, forthcomingness, connectedness, involvement, soft-heartedness, influenceability, empathy, caring behavior, unhindered compliance with easy-to-do requests, mutuality, and one-way affectionate love or warm feelings.

Researchers also have explored barriers to closeness and discovered multiple factors including defensive processes based on fear of vulnerability and abandonment (Firestone, R.W., & Firestone, L., 2004), as well as defensiveness, criticalness, contempt, and stonewalling (Gottman, 1999). ART offers factors that are antithetical to closeness including stonewalling, befuddling one's partner, dissociating, hardening of heart, being antidialogical, dominating the relationship, not being forthcoming, defendedness, self-centeredness, resisting talking, and resisting compliance with easy-to-do requests.

A more detailed discussion of each element that characterizes closeness is vital in providing therapists with an understanding of the value of closeness. Following are elements of these characteristics, along with case material as illustration of each.

- Openness. Openness involves the ability immediately and voluntarily to disclose one's own thoughts and feelings. For example, Marta came home from work and instead of becoming busy with household tasks, said immediately to her husband, Toby, "Something happened today that was very upsetting to me." Toby used Anthetic listening skills (discussed in Chapter 9) to listen to Marta, and they both felt close, she because she felt understood and accepted and he because he now knew Marta's state of mind. This process taught in ART is called *unwinding in your partner's arms*.

  Compare Marta's and Toby's interaction with Ilana and Mack, her husband. Ilana returned home from work and said, "I'm going to lie down." Mack said, "What's wrong?" She replied that nothing was wrong. Mack felt anxiety, because he knew she was feeling upset, but she was not disclosing why. He suspected she was upset with him but could not say it. He refrained from telling Ilana about his anxiety because he did not want to upset her. The partners were distant. That is, closeness had broken down because of each person's withdrawal. They were both following the precept in standard relationships of trying not to upset one's partner by talking about one's feelings.

Openness involves the willingness to talk about relevant information in oneself or about the other person. In other words, openness occurs when partners reveal feelings rather than withholding them and keeping them secret.

ART offers an explanation for the rationale for partners choosing withdrawal over openness. Despite conventional wisdom that partners offer in therapy for their withdrawal, such as, "I'm just a private person" or "I need time to unwind and gather myself together," ART clinical research indicates that a couple's withdrawal from each other results from an Inner Critic process in each partner. Self-disclosure triggers Inner Critic emotional punishments of shame and humiliation in the following ways. In Marta's and Toby's case, a habitual return from work pattern had plagued them and resulted in distance. Marta had previously reported in therapy one such moment. She had come home feeling tired and had absentmindedly kissed Toby, then gone to the bedroom to undress. Toby had followed her, sensing some distress. He asked her, "What's the matter?" Marta said, "Nothing's the matter; I'm just tired." Toby pressed, but Marta resisted and they ended the conversation angry at each other, with no resolution. During the ensuing session, the therapist helped them explore this process.

Therapist: When you look back at your feelings that day, Marta, would you say you were feeling more happy or unhappy about your day?

Marta: I'd have to say unhappy.

Therapist: Can you track back in your day when the unhappiness began?

Marta: Hmm. Well, now that I look back, I do remember that my co-worker said something insulting to me, and it stung. Then I couldn't come up with a response.

Therapist: What did you feel when you couldn't come up with a retort?

Marta: I felt embarrassed. Stupid. Humiliated.

Therapist: Can you see that those feelings of humiliation were a sign that your Inner Critic was pouncing, telling you that you should have a response and that not having one meant you were stupid?

Marta: Yes! I see that now. I didn't catch it then.

Therapist: Do you sense that you may have still been feeling some emotions from that encounter at the end of the day when you arrived home?

Marta: Definitely. I hadn't gotten to talk about it with anyone, and it was just sitting inside me.

Therapist: So, Toby, when Marta walked in the door, you sensed something in Marta?

Toby: Yes, I could tell something was troubling her. But I didn't know how to get her to tell me about it.

Therapist: Marta, did you know Toby was sensitive to you in that way?

Marta: No, I didn't. All I felt was I've got to get away from his questions.

Therapist: That's important. Feeling like you had to get away. What would you have felt if you had revealed what happened with your co-worker?

Marta: Shame. Toby would have seen that I couldn't come up with anything to say to that insult. I would have felt humiliated all over again.

Therapist: So, can you see that your Inner Critic not only pounced at the office but also at home with Toby, jolting you with feelings of shame and defectiveness.

Marta: Yes, I see that now.

Therapist: In order to get out from under those painful feelings, you tried to get away; to distance from Toby. Did that work?

Marta: No, in fact, it just added more pain, because then he and I were in a fight and felt distant all night. It was miserable.

Therapist: I want to offer you both a basic values choice to help you in the future with moments like this. Values are what we hold as important as a guide to our life. In this case, the values choice before you was closeness versus distance. Which would you like to choose?

Marta and Toby: Closeness. We want closeness.

Therapist: In order to achieve that closeness, you next must choose between openness and withdrawal. Openness means immediately and voluntarily sharing your feelings with each other. Openness is one key to creating closeness. Withdrawal, in which we withhold feelings from each other, creates distance. Which do you choose?

Marta: I want to learn to be open.

Toby: Me too. I would love to learn that.

Therapist: The key once you make that choice, is to get free from your Inner Critic, so you can be open.

Following this interchange, the therapist taught Toby and Marta Inner Critic challenging skills. As Toby and Marta practiced them at home, they were able to begin being open with each other about their feelings. They were able to practice unwinding in each other's arms. The therapist further taught them the skills of giving feedback when the other seemed distant, along with the skill of doing research rather than denying it (Chapter 5).

- Quotidian Honesty: A common pattern in modern society is the practice of quotidian dishonesty in which people refrain from telling each other the truth. For example, at Christmas, it is frequent practice for people to say upon unwrapping a gift, "Oh! It's just what I wanted!" even though the gift is not to their taste or liking. The ART understanding of this process is that such dishonesty is an attempt to avoid guilt about hurting the feelings of the giver. Were the recipient to be honest, his or her Inner Critic would plead them guilty of rudeness, even were the recipient to be honest in a caring way. Such dishonesty creates walls of distance, which may be acceptable if the people do not want closeness. However, even those who desire closeness, particularly life partners, practice quotidian dishonesty, not realizing the toll it takes in loss of closeness.

  In order to create the closeness of an HVR, partners will need to choose Quotidian Honesty, in which they practice truth-telling. An important note the therapist must clarify for partners is that quotidian honesty must be distinguished from saying anything, using any tone of voice. Nor does it equate with acting out blaming, judgmentalism, anger, or other forms of negativity. Any negative feelings are to be reported in a neutral manner; for example, "I feel an impulse to be judgmental." Acted-out feelings result in the pain common in an LVR in contrast to reporting feelings essential to HVRs. Another example of quotidian honesty is the ability to say "No." For example, "I don't want to go on vacation where you want to go. Let's negotiate a place we'll both enjoy."
- Being Forthcoming: This element is essentially about self-disclosure.

  Self-disclosure means talking about oneself; reporting feelings and opinions; expressing thoughts; declaring who one is; revealing likes and dislikes; talking about what is happening in one's life; describing current projects and activities; and announcing hopes and plans.

  The opposite of being forthcoming includes remaining silent in order to not reveal feelings or thoughts and telling a partial truth. It inevitably involves withholding something important from one's partner. For example, when one partner asks the other, "Where will we have lunch? How about a burger?" and the other replies, "That's okay" rather than expressing a genuine response, which might be, "I want to go to that new restaurant we talked about."

From an ART perspective, the Inner Critic is instrumental in such lack of forthcomingness, in that were partners to fully volunteer their feelings, the Inner Critic would condemn them for being rude and inflict a jolt of guilt.

- Connectedness: This element refers to the ability to respond *directly* and appropriately to a remark. It involves responding without tangentializing, following the speaker's agenda without imposing one's own. When the initiator asks a question, a direct response might be an actual answer to the question, or it might be, "I'd rather not answer that question."

  The opposite of connectedness is disconnectedness, where no direct response is given. Again the Inner Critic is implicated in that were the person to answer in a connected way, the Inner Critic would inflict painful feelings of humiliation or guilt. The result is inevitably low-voltage communication.
- Involvement: Partners who choose a low-voltage pattern are willing to accept what might be called "mere contact." They do not desire a lot of involvement and may even feel scared of the closeness that comes with such involvement.

  High-voltage partners, on the other hand, want the intensity of involvement even if it feels scary.

  Involvement overlaps some of the other categories mentioned in this chapter, since it includes giving and receiving feedback, being self-disclosing, and wanting to know what the other person is thinking and feeling. However, the most important feature of involvement is the desire and ability to respond in depth to what the other has said rather than being silent. It involves coming to grips with what the partner says instead of producing a cliché or responding only partially.

  An important distinction exists between connection and involvement. Connection is merely a direct response. For example, a connected response to the question, "What are you feeling right now?" might be, "I'd rather not talk about my feelings." An involved response would comprise connection along with more depth of information. For example to the previous question, an involved answer might be, "I'm feeling relaxed, happy to have this time with you, but a little awkward because we haven't spent much time together." (A disconnected response might be as follows: "Oh, everybody's talking about feelings nowadays.")
- Soft-heartedness: It refers to loving-kindness, warmth, compassion, being understanding, gentleness, considerateness, benevolence, having goodwill toward a person, giving the benefit of the doubt, and generosity. It is a value that is essential for a successful HVR, an ideal toward which the couple may work.

  In contrast, hard-heartedness is best described as a general demeanor of toughness, harshness, spitefulness, meanness, guardedness, premature contentiousness, petulance, surliness, bristliness, coldness, abrasiveness, suspiciousness, insensitivity, sulkiness, self-centeredness, holding a grudge, scowling, and appearing sullen. Persons who hold hard-heartedness as a defense from which they live, will not be able to produce an HVR for an obvious reason: The pain of being close to a hard-hearted person is too severe to sustain intimacy.

In reviewing polar types, it becomes evident that persons who are Tough polar types have a hard time being soft-hearted. Persons who are Tender tend to relate in a soft-hearted manner automatically.

- Influenceability: Research definitively points to the vital importance of couple's ability to accept influence from each other (Gottman, 1999). In ART, influenceability refers to being influenced by the wishes and requests of one's partner. Requisite in having influenceability is a general receptivity toward what one's partner says. For example, if one partner says to the other, "I'm scared of you," a non-receptive response would be, "I don't believe you" or "Why should you be scared of me" or even "You have no reason to be scared of me." A receptive, influenceable response would be "Tell me more about that."

  In an additional example, a partner says, "You seem to be angry." An influenceable response would be, "Can you tell me what leads you to say that?" Non-influenceable responses would include, "No, I'm not" and "You're the one who's angry."

  It is important to state here that ART does not hold that a partner must validate what the other says, which would imply supporting the truth or validity of an assertion. Influenceability instead refers to being open to the other by doing Research (Chapter 12) and by being provisional in any position one holds.
- Empathizing: Researchers agree that the element of empathizing is essential for closeness, since it involves understanding what each other is feeling. This is best achieved by partners imagining themselves inside the mind of the other and asking themselves what thoughts and feelings might he or she be having. It requires giving up self-centeredness in favor of attending to the other. However, partners may experience blocks to empathizing in the form of Inner Critic propaganda that attending to one's partner is humiliating, implying that one is inferior when not the center of attention.

Value 4: Positivity

The destructive impact of negativity on relationships is undeniable. John Gottman's term, "corrosive," is telling, in that his research clearly revealed that negative relating through criticism, defensiveness, contempt, and stonewalling (Gottman's *Four Horsemen of the Apocalypse*) lead not only to unhappy marriages but almost inevitably to divorce (Gottman, 1994; Gottman, 1999). Prior to dissolution of a marriage, such negativity leads couples to try to manage their distress through emotional disengagement; what Gottman calls the *Distance and Isolation Cascade.* From an ART perspective, such a pattern of distance and isolating can be described as an LVR.

In contrast, marital stability and even outcome, Gottman found, could be predicted from the ratio of positivity to negativity (five positives to one negative). Anthetic Relationship Therapy seeks to offer couples not merely marital stability, but rather the goal of optimality. In order to achieve optimal, that is, high-voltage relating, a couple's ability to hold positivity as a guiding value is essential. In fact, the Anthetic therapist encourages a 10:1 ratio of positivity to negativity and offers both intrapersonal as well as interpersonal skills for increasing positivity (Chapter 9).

Value 5: Using the Relationship for Psychological Growth

Perhaps the most important value that distinguishes LVRs from HVRs is that couples aspiring to high-voltage relating choose to use their relationship for each partner's psychological growth. In contrast, low-voltage partners are frequently guided by maintaining equilibrium and avoiding addressing conflict. They do not value doing the work of psychological processing, insight seeking, and transformative change.

Anthetic Relationship Therapy offers couples a step-by-step Anthetic Growth Process, facilitating their movement from desire for closeness to a values choice for closeness to Inner Freedom. The steps proceed as follows:

Step 1

The couple indicates to the therapist a desire for closeness. Pip and Rob, ages 47 and 38, sought help for a newly developing depth in their relationship. At the first session, Pip revealed, "We've known each other casually for a couple years, but about six months ago we realized we were attracted to each other in a more romantic way. We started seeing each other and then decided to move in together."

Rob added, "Yes, we thought we'd take it slow, so although we're having an intimate sexual relationship, we each decided to have our own bedroom."

Pip went on to add, "And that's what led us to call you. I had surgery about eight months ago with some complications. It sort of got me in touch with my mortality. So, I asked Rob, 'If I'm ever not awake (I'm the early riser) when you get up, would you come and check on me, just to make sure I'm breathing or haven't had a stroke or something?' He said ok; he would. Well, last week I was working on a project at work that left me exhausted. I went to bed at the usual time but slept late. When Rob got up before I did, he came in my room (I was just sitting up in bed) and said, 'Ya still breathin'? I felt a sting, kind of confused, like, well he just did what I asked but it felt like he was angry at me or hostile as he did it. We've been sort of distant since then, and I don't want this to fester. So, I asked him if he'd come with me to counseling, and he agreed."

Rob nodded, "Yeah, I don't understand what happened and why Pip has backed away from me. I want us to move forward, not back."

At this point, the therapist through empathic doubling (Chapter 10), offered, "Is it like, 'We're wanting more closeness, but we're puzzled because instead we're getting more distant. And we're thinking the distance began with that morning check?"

Both men nodded and said, "Yes, that's exactly it."

In this presentation of their issue, both indicated a desire for closeness.

Step 2: Values Choice

The therapist then articulates the values choice and offers the couple the opportunity to make their choice explicit. She says, "So, in terms of what you value and what you want to guide your relationship, it sounds like you want closeness instead of distance." (The couple nods as she talks.) She guides them, "If it fits, would you turn to each other and state, 'I choose closeness in our relationship.'"

Rob and Pip turned toward each other, smiled, spontaneously grabbed each other's hands and said, "I choose closeness in our relationship."

By offering the couple the opportunity to explicitly state their values choice, the therapist fosters the grounding connection as well as an intensification of the voltage between them.

Step 3: Processing Blocks to Living out the Values Choice

Once the therapist and couple have established the guiding value the couple desires, identifying and processing any blocks to the value follows. In this case, the value of closeness is being prevented from being actualized in their relationship. The couple is puzzled, since in their own minds and in their stated choice, each clearly wants closeness. The therapist helps the couple identify and process blocks either has, that is, explore toward understanding and becoming free from the block.

The therapist explains, "Because you both so clearly want closeness in your relationship and are puzzled that distance is occurring, you can infer that some psychological block in either or both of you is surfacing and preventing closeness." She offers a verbal contract for processing. "Would you like my help in identifying the blocks and getting free from their contaminating your closeness?" Both partners nod emphatically and say, "Absolutely!"

The therapist continues, "Let's back up a bit to what led to your pain, Pip. You mentioned that you had felt vulnerable about your mortality since your surgery and had made a request of Rob that he check on you if you were not up in the morning at your usual earlier time of rising." (Pip nods.) "You, Rob, had agreed to the request." (Rob says, "Yes.") "So, Rob, tell me if I have this right. When Pip was not awake at his normal time, you remembered that you had agreed to check on him and went into his room to do so." (Rob assents, "That's right.") Continuing, the therapist states, "When you saw Pip sitting up, you asked, 'Ya' breathin'?' at which point, you, Pip, felt a twinge of pain. Is that right?"

Pip says, "Yes, exactly."

"Can you say more, Pip, about the twinge of pain?"

Pip thinks and says, "It felt like Rob was angry or even sort of hostile. Like he was doing something he really didn't want to be doing."

The therapist asks Rob, "Were you aware of feeling any anger or hostile feelings, Rob?"

Rob thinks and says, "Not at the time, but as we're talking about it, I can get a sense that my tone was sort of angry."

Some important psychoeducation appears necessary at this point, so the therapist explains, "This was an important moment I want to point out so you can start catching these. When we have agreed to do a request but find that we fulfill the request with some anger or resistance, it's a clue that we are not freely complying. Something; that is, some internal process is leading to the feelings of anger." Both men listen and nod.

"I want to give you each skills for handling such a moment. First, I want to give you the skills of *Offering Feedback* and of *Using Feedback for Growth*. In this instance, you, Pip, can Offer Feedback and you, Rob, can use the Feedback for Growth. Pip, Offering Feedback involves feeling the twinge of pain which indicates Rob may have been having some anger and then asking him, 'Were you feeling angry when you checked on me?' So, would you like to ask Rob that now?"

Pip laughed a bit nervously but turned to Rob and asked, "Were you feeling angry when you checked on me?"

The therapist then instructs Rob, "Rob, the skill of Using Feedback for Growth involves considering the feedback you get, exploring inwardly to see if some feeling is keeping you from being free. By that I mean, if you were free and not blocked, you would either say, 'No, I don't want to check on Pip. I don't care about him in that way.' Or you would say, 'No, I don't want to check on Pip; although I care about him, I don't have that to give,' or 'I want to check on Pip, because I care about him, and I am happy to do that.'"

Rob, considering this says, "As I think about what you're saying, I think, 'I do care about Pip and I do have that to give.' So now, I'm puzzled that for some reason I wasn't happy to do it that day."

The therapist comments, "What you just said is an example of the ideal attitude to have toward considering feedback, Rob, that is, curiosity about your inner workings. You reflected on what you felt; discovered that you really did have caring toward Pip; and then noted that you felt puzzled that your attitude didn't get communicated to Pip. Now, you are curious, wondering why you weren't happy to do what you really wanted to do."

"Now I want to give you another skill for Using Feedback for Growth. It's a self-reflection skill that consists of an incomplete sentence to complete in order to explore what is underneath any behavior that puzzles you. It goes like this, 'I don't want to check on you Pip, because. . . .' Would you be willing to try this?"

Rob says, "Yes. I don't want to check on you Pip, because. . .Hmm. . .because it's so weak of you to want me to check on you. Huh! I didn't know I felt that. But, I do. I don't ask anybody to check on me, because that would be childish, babyish."

The therapist was then able to lead Rob into understanding that the Inner Critic and prototype had installed shoulds which were driving his feelings of contempt toward weakness. Rob was able to challenge the Inner Critic shoulds which had led to some polar type rigidity and was able to add more tenderness to his repertoire. Closeness between the partners increased.

HELPING A COUPLE WITH VALUES CHOICE

Before the therapist can teach skills to a couple, he or she must listen for and articulate what values are guiding the partners. When couples come to therapy, quite often the values by which they are living are tacit and unconscious. The therapist can help them become conscious of their values by teaching them the concept of values choice; then helping the couple consciously choose the values they want in their relationship and articulate it to each other.

Anthetic Relationship Therapy offers therapists a protocol for examining and articulating a couple's values. Following is the ART *Values Choice Intervention*:

The therapist begins with, "Before we go farther, I want to lay out a concept that is fundamental to going forward. It is the concept of values choice. A value is something we hold as important and that we guide our lives by. For example, we can choose a combat marriage or a loving marriage. A combat marriage is one in which partners value escalating conflict through acting out their negative feelings. A loving marriage is one in which partners are guided by warm feelings and good will toward each other."

"So, I want to ask you: Do you choose a combat marriage or a loving marriage?"

Once the partners individually state to the therapist their values choice, the therapist asks them to turn to each other and declare their choice.

In each case, the therapist perceives through the couple's expressions of distress which values choice is implied. Then the therapist presents the values choice as a dichotomy. In the previous intervention, the therapist offered the combat marriage/loving marriage dichotomy. Given other issues exhibited by the couple, she might offer dichotomies of distance versus closeness; positivity versus negativity; or psychological growth versus business as usual. Establishing the guiding value orients couples to what is important and provides a ground from which to plan interventions toward actualizing the value.

Chapter 6

Eight Intrapersonal High-Voltage Skills

In equipping couples toward optimal relating, Anthetic Relationship Therapy takes the perspective that the intrapersonal world of each partner is instrumental in how each relates to the other. What becomes enacted on the conscious stage of their relationship has roots in the subconscious of each partner. Previous theorists have pioneered the intrapsychic perspective as applied to couples and families, including Satir, (1978), Scharff, D., & Scharff, J. (1987), and Schwartz (1995) and offered credence to the importance of addressing psychological blocks in partners in order to reduce couple distress and increase competence for intimate relating. Satir's contribution on increasing self-esteem through self-awareness of internal functioning laid groundwork for intrapsychic work. Scharff & Scharff's work on internalized objects had as its goal increased insight of family members in order to deal with family distress. Schwartz's work on internal family systems has as its goal to collaboratively equip family members to identify and work with internal parts in order to deal with distress.

Anthetic Relationship Theory offers a new archetype having as its goal optimality, rather than relief of couple distress. In addition, the approach holds that in order to achieve optimal relating, partners must possess skills for their own psychological growth. These internal or intrapsychic skills are essential in creating the infrastructure to support optimal relating skills. This chapter lays the groundwork for intrapsychic work through skills to prepare each partner to work with his or her emerging internal world.

Slowing Down, Relaxing, and Self-Soothing

The intensity of intimate relationships creates conditions for mixtures of powerful emotions culminating in a physiological state of *diffuse physiological arousal* in partners (Gottman, 1999). When in this state of sympathetic nervous system activation, partners experience reduced ability to listen and attend to one another, to process information, and to access new learning. An essential task of therapy is to equip couples with skills for both self-soothing and partner-soothing in order to counter the psychological and interpersonal effects of this process.

Anthetic Relationship Therapy proceeds into the intrapsychic world of each partner in an orderly fashion. In order to help partners identify a state of diffuse physiological arousal, the therapist teaches them to recognize two clues. The first clue occurs as the partner engages in Frantic Talk. Tense and high-strung like a spirited race horse in the starting gate, the person is quick to respond with kneejerk reactions. He or she finds it difficult to take time to think and reflect before speaking. In this state, the frantic partner interrupts the other frequently and has difficulty being interrupted. The second clue is revealed as the person in this state may be angry or indignant. He or she is especially quick to defend himself or herself instead of researching and carefully considering any feedback received. The person is apt to respond from the Reactive Self, not the Executive Self. In short, driven by a should to react quickly, the person enters a state of mind where there is no time for processing nor for reflective reasoning.

The skill of *slowing down* gives the person time to engage in processing. The therapist teaches the partner first to come to an abrupt halt paired with a deliberate decision to appropriate psychological space to process. The following releasing statements may be used, including, "I have the right to take my time. I have the right to think before I speak. And I have the right to postpone speaking as long as I want. Several minutes. Or hours. Perhaps a full day. Or several days. Or even longer."

In addition, the therapist may teach partners a technique drawn from Recovery, Inc. (Low, 1950). When a person becomes reactive, Recovery offers the concept of *working yourself up.* Anthetic Relationship Therapy defines the concept using the following indicators: a strident voice, anger, defensiveness, judgmentalism, frozenness, and other automatic reactions. In order to counter this process, Recovery uses the term *work yourself down.* This involves soothing oneself through calming self-statements such as, "This isn't the end of the world"; "This isn't a tragedy"; and "This too will pass."

The third technique therapists may teach directly addresses the body tension involved in diffuse physiological arousal, that is the skill of relaxing. To relax, the therapist instructs the person to first close his or her eyes whenever this occurs; even when someone is talking to him or her. The person then tells his or her partner, "I need to relax now." Following this, the person looks inside and relaxes each tense spot in the body. The process involves saying to oneself: "Feel the tension in your eyes and forehead. Let your facial muscles relax. Each time you exhale, let a wave of relaxation flow downward through your whole body. Your face is feeling heavy and warm. The relaxation is moving through your shoulders, down through your chest, your arms and hands, your pelvis, your legs and feet. Now your whole body is feeling very heavy and warm. You are relaxing parts of your body that you haven't relaxed in a long, long time. Now just be with your relaxed body for as long as you want. When you're ready, open your eyes and come back to the place you're in." (The therapist can provide a tape of these statements for partners to play or alternatively, may suggest partners make a tape of their own voices.) In the relaxed state that ensues, partners are ready to engage in cognitive and emotional processing.

Making a Value Shift

The HVR cannot be achieved through sheer willpower. The reason for this is that any action in which partners engage is always preceded by a value. If partners learn Inner Critic challenging, they do so because they value inner freedom and Anthetic growth. If they do not want to learn it, they do so because they value reactive living. In order to work toward creating an HVR, partners must first make a number of value shifts. The values lay the foundation as support the high-voltage skills.

Following is the six-step protocol the therapist teaches the couple to use whenever a value shift is indicated:

- First, begin with the value the person presently holds. The person then reflects on the past to discover where and when he or she learned the value and from whom. For example, if the partner holds the value of politeness and not upsetting the partner, he or she may reflect, "What I learned from you, Mom, was 'Don't upset your father. Don't tell him you didn't like the restaurant he took us to. That would hurt his feelings. Instead, put on your politeness face. Don't be honest.'"
- Second, guide the person to make a list of the advantages and disadvantages of continuing to be guided by the old value when talking to the partner. If the partner invites him or her to a restaurant, one advantage of being guided by the politeness value is that the partner will not get upset. A disadvantage is that the partner may invite the person to go to the same restaurant again and again, mistakenly thinking he or she is doing what pleases the person.
- Third, the therapist helps the person examine the new value he or she is considering. Take, for example, Quotidian Honesty. List the advantages and disadvantages of holding the new value. One disadvantage of quotidian honesty might be that one's partner would feel upset, hurt and perhaps

angry if the person revealed that he or she did not like something the partner did. In other words, honesty would have repercussions. On the other hand, an advantage of quotidian honesty is that the partners would know each other's preferences in greater depth and thus would create emotional closeness.

- In order to handle possible repercussions of quotidian honesty, the therapist can assist the partners to make an agreement to be honest about likes, dislikes, and feelings. Then the therapist helps each partner agree to work on any hurt feelings that might arise from honesty.
- Fourth, the partners decide which value is best for the type of relationship they desire. In the case of quotidian honesty, a choice for this value would produce the emotional closeness of an HVR. A choice to prioritize politeness would produce less closeness and an LVR. Each has its advantages and disadvantages and is a free choice of the partners.
- Fifth, the therapist assists partners in eliminating any Inner Critic shoulds that might influence their decision, so the choice will not be based on shoulds.
- Finally, the therapist asks the partners to distill the previous steps into a decision regarding which value by which they choose to live. The therapist helps them declare the choice to each other.
- Once couples learn the skill of values testing, they can use it to analyze and evaluate any of the values that might be either sabotaging or supporting their psychological growth work toward an HVR.

Introspecting: The Anthetic Archeology of Reactive Structures

Introspecting involves looking within; turning one's attention away from the external world and looking into one's inner world. By doing so, a partner can perceive his or her thoughts, feelings, impulses, images, and attitudes. This skill is essential for doing Anthetic Self-Analysis and answering why-questions; for example, "Why am I afraid of my partner?" "Why am I being defensive?" and "Why am I being judgmental?" The skill is required for discovering the subconscious elements that may be driving the reactive behavior that is preventing the partner from creating an HVR.

This skill must first be preceded by the skill of slowing down and relaxing. Then the therapist teaches partners to look inside and become aware of what bubbles up from their subconscious minds, accepting any thoughts or feelings or impulses and just noting them. The ability to simply note the feelings may be achieved by addressing any self-criticalness regarding any element with Inner Critic challenging. Once any Inner Critic condemnation is eliminated, what will remain will be curiosity that motivates task-oriented Introspecting.

The goal of introspecting is to identify any reactivity that would result in an impediment to optimal relating.

Reactive Self-Structure is a term used in Anthetic Therapy to refer to the internal psychological structures created by the psyche in reaction to the threat of emotional punishment by the Inner Critic (Elliott, J., & Elliott, K., 2000, p. 76). The structure includes patterns of feelings, thoughts, decisions, and impulses created as a way of coping with pain. However, the reactive self-structure is responsible for the major reactive themes in a person's life. Examples of major reactive themes include self-disempowerment, victim stance, characterological anger, as well as each rigid polar type.

Anthetic Therapy sees each Reactive Self-Structure not as a terminal trait but rather as an opportunity for further inner freedom and growth. The Anthetic Therapy protocol for helping a person work toward more freedom can be seen as akin to an archeological dig; carefully unearthing layer by layer of material in order to reveal underlying elements. Some of these elements are fragments of structure pointing to the pure gold of natural self possibilities that have been submerged. The process moves from what may be ego-dystonic material of which the person is consciously aware down through deeper and deeper subconscious material which is either ego-syntonic or unconscious to the individual. The following seven-step protocol first is introduced to the couple by the therapist and then is provided as a handout to be used by them outside of sessions.

- Step 1: Uncovering Rules about the Reactivity. Take the case of Layla, who explored The Structure of Learned Disempowerment, an ego-dystonic problem that surfaced in her relationship with Paolo. The therapist elicited such rules using the WILFY dialogue (Elliott, K.J., 1995), but could have also done so through talk therapy. Because rules for living are often ego-dystonic, the person frequently can access these consciously. In the example of Layla, the rules she had learned included, "Never ask for help."
- Step 2: Uncovering Messages that Negate the Natural Self. Partners function optimally when their Natural Self impulses toward need fulfillment have been supported throughout their development. However, partners who have not had such support, often exhibit a lack of assertiveness secondary to having received messages throughout their lives that negate the Natural Self. Anthetic Relationship Therapy elicits such messages through Anthetic Dialogue or through traditional talk therapy. In Layla's case, the therapist directed her to sit in an empty chair and speak from the prototype that had instilled the messages; in this case, she had identified as her father. Messages included, "You don't need help. You don't deserve help. You're a girl; you're not worthy of my help. To be Male is ok; to be Female is not ok."

- Step 3: "Your Purpose" Messages that Negate the Natural Self. At this point in the protocol, the therapist helps the person sharpen the elicitation of internalized messages by offering the sentence stem, "Your purpose is to ___________." Layla's Anthetic Dialogue with her father revealed messages consisting of, "Your purpose is to build up my male ego. A female's only worth is to build up a male."
- Step 4: Learned Consequences. Having elicited the specific messages of negation of the Natural Self, the therapist now helps the person continue to dialogue with the prototype in order to identify the impact of the learning carried from the prototype by offering the incomplete sentence, "I learned that if I did not live according to your philosophy, the consequences to me would be ___________." In the example of Layla, the therapist directed her to return to her original chair and speak to the prototype, her father, as imagined in the previous chair. She completed the sentence stem with, "I learned if I didn't live by your philosophy, the consequences were abandonment, criticism, punishment, and watching others receive what I wasn't given."
- Step 5: Revealing the Coping Structure Developed to Deal with the Pain. Typically, in order to deal with the pain the person experienced, he or she has developed a compensatory or defensive structure. The therapist prompts the person to continue the dialogue with the prototype with the following sentence stem, "To deal with this pain, I __________." Layla responded, "To deal with this pain, I became a wallflower, an ornament, a trophy. I was your ornament, Dad, and I was my first husband's trophy wife. Now, with Paolo, I'm trying to change this pattern, but I find myself not telling him what I want or need, just like I learned to do with you."
- Step 6: Life Reclaimed. As the person psychologically walks through the force field of the propaganda revealed in the above archeological process, catharsis will usually have occurred. At this point, the therapist guides the person to the gold of the Natural Self and assists him or her in reclaiming it, that is welcomes it and the implications for living and relating. The therapist uses an Anthetic Double along with sentence stems: "From now on, I reclaim that ____________." Layla completed the sentence with, "I can just ask for a want or a need to be met. I claim that there aren't any rules for help. I have the right to ask for help any time I like." In order to actualize this decision in her relationship with Paolo, the therapist prompted Layla, "Would you turn to Paolo and tell him that?" Following her declaration to Paolo, he nodded, reached for her hand, and said, "Yes, you do. I want you to tell me your wants and needs. I am here to help you." If a partner does not volunteer a response as Paolo did, the therapist can ask the partner to respond. As a further strengthening of the person's life reclamation, the therapist can encourage him or her to identify images such as inner figures, archetypes, and symbols to represent the change. Layla had been drawn to

a painting of Venus and chose to print a copy off the internet and post it in prominent places where she could have a visual reminder of her declaration.

- Step 7: Behavior Change. The final step in this process involves a discussion by the therapist and client to identify opportunities for actualizing in everyday behavior this reclaimed option. The format follows the structure, "I am going to ask for help from _______ about __________." Layla determined that she was going to ask Paolo for help with setting boundaries with her father, who expected her to prioritize taking his calls, even when she was busy. The therapist helped her to ask for this in the session. In addition, because she had developed a pattern of never buying anything for herself, Layla asked Paolo to support her in using a portion of the money she earned to buy items that gave her pleasure.

Self-Monitoring

Moment-by-moment *self-monitoring* is a more systematic form of introspection, consisting of three parts: First, the person takes a step back from his or her thoughts, feelings, and impulses and simply observes them. The person may note, "Am I feeling anger?" Then the therapist guides to just step back from the anger psychologically and just observe it. This process is repeated for fear, Inner Critic messages, defensiveness, judgmentalism, and impulses to punish one's partner or to withdraw or to pretend to knowledge one does not possess. The process essentially involves bracketing everything in one's psyche, temporarily putting it out of play while taking a look at it. The therapist may find it helpful to offer the metaphor of the Jukebox Process in which one functions like a jukebox. To explain, when someone pushes one of the person's buttons, he or she has no choice but to play a pre-set tune. The tune perhaps is "I'll get revenge by withdrawing" or "I have a compulsion to get acquitted by defending myself." As the person identifies elements of automaticity, he or she moves in the direction of inner freedom. For some individuals, a should to be spontaneous may present a psychological block to practicing this step. In such cases, the therapist may guide the person to make a releasing statement to take back his or her right to be easygoing, slow-paced, and deliberate.

The second step involves evaluating what one is about to say or do. In addition, the person reflects on whether to do so would be consistent with his or her values, factually correct, rational, reactive, constructive or destructive to the relationship, helpful or injurious.

In light of the reflection in the second step, the person decides what to do and then does it refrains from doing it in the third step. In the case of a decision to refrain, the person may find giving a Pull Report helpful; for example, "I feel a pull to defend myself, but I'm not going to go there."

As partners engage in self-monitoring, they shift from being reactively at the mercy of impulses and feelings to functioning from their Executive Selves, that is, in charge of their lives. The therapist can encourage them that practice of this skill will lead to it becoming second nature as well as pleasurable.

Disrupting Trances and Machine-like Behavior

The importance of identifying underlying emotions has been a central theme in couple approaches such as Emotionally Focused Couple Therapy (Greenberg & Johnson, 1988). In addition, a number of psychodynamic couple approaches have incorporated a core therapeutic goal of bringing subconscious material to conscious awareness in order to reverse the negative effect on relationships such material frequently produces (Firestone & Catlett, 2001; Scharff & Scharff, 1991). Anthetic Relationship Therapy agrees with this basic premise and holds that in order to create an HVR, partners must work toward becoming free from the subconscious machinery that tends to drive them.

In order to equip couples to identify subconsciously driven behavior, the therapist must teach a fundamental distinction. Behavior that is freely chosen and under executive self control is easily interruptible. Driven behavior is not. A clue that a person is engaging in machinelike behavior involves the statement, "That's just the way I am." This statement indicates an ego-syntonic position in which the person is unaware of underlying motivations, thoughts, and feelings. Take the case of Jed, who displayed an acquittal trance when his wife, Stefanie, made a request:

STEFANIE: "Jed, I have a request that you spend more time with the kids."

JED: "What are you talking about? You know I love those kids. That's why I work so late every night: to buy them clothes and the things they need. I pay for ballet lessons for Sharon and guitar lessons for Jacob."

The therapist helped Jed explore his automatic response using the Jukebox Metaphor. Reflection revealed that Jed's jukebox was playing, "Defend yourself. Don't do Research. Don't try to discover what your partner means." The therapist then helped Jed slow down, relax, and ask Stefanie what she had meant. She clarified that she did not want him to prioritize money but rather that the children have a daddy to spend time with them.

Following are three reflective-delay skills taught in Anthetic Relationship Therapy to help partners disrupt the machinelike behavior that prevents the achievement of the HVR:

1. "I don't have to defend myself." This position statement, voiced out loud, disrupted Jed's spontaneous dysfunctionality and permitted him to reflect on what was happening. When he made this releasing statement, he was able to choose a different option and engage in Research, including asking Stefanie, "Can you tell me more about that?"
2. "Hey! Wait a minute!" When said to oneself or out loud to one's partner, this exclamation disrupts machinelike behavior by providing psychological space in which to think and reflect. It also helps a person slow down and relax and is useful when a person feels the pull of a compulsion.
3. "Let me think about it and get back to you." At first glance, this may look like a request for permission; however, it is not. Rather, it is a position statement that disrupts the machinery that compels a person to respond immediately and unreflectively to feedback or to a request.

Revising Dysfunctional Learnings

Personality and social psychology research point to the role of cognition and affect in interdependent relationships. Humans naturally function in the world of relationships with one another by developing habitual tendencies to recognize common features of situations and people and then to respond in specific ways that are a complex of their own needs, partner's needs, and outcome implications of an interaction (Cosmides & Tooby, 1992; Kelley, 1979, 1997; Rusbult, Kumashiro, Coolsen, & Kirchner, 2004). Conclusions that humans draw from this process may constitute prosocial, asocial, or antisocial rules for relating. Anthetic Relationship Therapy offers the term *Cherished Dysfunctional Beliefs* for rules that hinder closeness; those that function like ghosts from the past, haunting the person's present thoughts, feelings, attitudes, and behavior. Examples of such beliefs are, "Be sensitive and helpful to people, and they'll be nice to you, which will reduce your pain" associated with the Tender polar type; "Dominate people, and you can make them do what you want, which will reduce your pain" adopted by the Tough polar type; "Withdraw from people and scale down your needs, which will reduce your pain" held by the Self-Sufficient polar type; and "Be self-effacing and dependent on people's approval, and they won't criticize you, which will reduce your pain" associated with the Tender-Dependent polar type.

From a psychodynamic perspective, each of the above strategies is essentially an anesthetic for the Inner Critic's emotional punishments, that is, an attempt to reduce pain engendered by the Inner Critic. The term *cherished* regarding dysfunctional beliefs is drawn from the rigid reliance a person places upon guiding behavior by the beliefs, because the beliefs have been the only reliable pain relief they have achieved. Despite their value for pain relief, at the point of presentation in therapy, the partners have inevitably experienced a significant amount of negative sequelae from living by the beliefs.

As mentioned in Chapter 2, Anthetic Therapy is based on a learning model, not a trauma model (Elliott, J.E, 1992b; Elliott, K.J., 1995); Elliott, K.J., 1999). That is, this approach holds that it is not always the trauma itself that causes problems in adult life but rather what the person learns from it. However, the trauma may have produced frozen feelings that have locked in the learnings. If this has happened, the feelings may need to be thawed and loosened through catharsis so they are no longer impedimental. When this thawing occurs, the dysfunctional learnings can become accessible and now open to revision. In order to help couples discover their Cherished Dysfunctional Beliefs, the therapist guides the person in engaging in unearthing work by engaging in Anthetic Dialogue with people from their past who might have been the occasions of the adoption of the Cherished Dysfunction Belief.

Consider the case of Jill, who was unable to connect with her husband Nolan. "She won't answer my questions," Nolan told the therapist. "She says things like 'I'm having a lot of problems at work,' and I'll ask her what problems, and she says 'Oh, I don't want to go into it.' But then she's all moody and touchy. Remote and withdrawn. Unavailable."

As the therapist worked with Jill using Anthetic Dialogue and the anthetic archeology of reactive self-structure, what emerged was a pattern of fear of feeling humiliated by her supervisor. She reported that the fear was so severe she had even thought, "If I can't do my job well, why do I go on living? I might as well commit suicide." (The therapist assessed Jill's suicide risk and found that she would never do it for a number of reasons.)

In talking about her childhood, Jill revealed that when she was in the fourth grade, her father, who previously had been doting on her, tried to tutor her in arithmetic. He became frustrated with her difficulty in understanding new concepts and began scolding her when she could not learn quickly enough. The scolding represented a shift in their relationship that comprised a loss of closeness and doting Jill had previously enjoyed. "Daddy used to ask me if I understood what he was teaching me," she said, "and I was so afraid of him, I said yes, even when I didn't. Now when Nolan asks me a question, I don't want to show how bad I am by giving him the wrong answer. So I don't say anything. I want to protect myself."

Jill's cherished dysfunctional belief was "don't respond if your answer will be humiliating." The therapist directed her in Anthetic Dialogue, and she was able to express and thaw the frozen feelings of anger and just beneath the anger, some pain. As soon as she did this, she was able to do Inner Critic challenging; for example, "I have the right not to know the answer" and "I have the right to feel humiliated. It's just a feeling, not a fact. It's something my Inner Critic is telling me. And it's not the end of the world. I've felt humiliated before, and I survived just fine, and if I feel humiliated again, I'll survive again."

The therapist then encouraged Jill to *welcome* feelings of humiliation. "Welcome humiliation?" Jill was nonplussed. "Why in the world should I do that?" The therapist explained that welcoming humiliation would help her desensitize to those feelings. In addition, feelings of humiliation could be an important indicator that she was feeling reluctant to tell the truth and a signal that she may be holding back from asserting herself with Nolan.

"Hmm," she said, "I see what you're saying." Jill was able to learn to desensitize to humiliation, which enabled her to engage in an involved conversation with her husband.

In order to help partners spot Cherished Dysfunctional Beliefs such as Jill did, the therapist helps the person welcome feedback about his or her behavior that indicate clues that such a belief is operating. During this process, the therapist will assist with listening nondefensively and challenging any Inner Critic shoulds that surface. Some possible feedback that may be offered include, "Are you feeling defensive?" "You seem distant"; "Are you feeling judgmental?" "Did your Inner Critic just pounce?" and "Are you in your Little Boy (or Little Girl)?" Once the person explores this feedback, he or she can spot any dysfunctional learning through Anthetic Dialogue with inner figures from the past, as the learning will have its source in such introjects.

Disengaging and Bracketing

Reactivity occurs when a person fuses with the elements in the psyche. Anthetic Dialogue is the method of choice for disengaging from those fusions and bracketing them. Although the process of Anthetic Dialogue itself can result in a certain amount of disengagement, special techniques are needed for the complete disengagement required for individuation. In addition to disengaging from the element, the person also must reflect on it and make a redecision about it.

However, the fusion may be so thoroughgoing in a person that he or she is unaware that it exists. The therapist can help the person recognize the reactivity of these fusions by four criteria: (a) Does the person feel an emotional pull toward the element? (b) Does the person express indignation when someone challenges him or her about the element? (c) Does the person feel a strange reluctance to evaluate the element rationally? and (d) Is there a driven, impulsive quality to his or her decisions and resulting behavior, such that it is difficult or impossible to interrupt them?

Inner compulsivity is evidenced when a person chooses one item impulsively without making a survey of all the available items. Inner freedom, on the other hand, is reflective freedom. It is displayed when the person surveys all the possibilities before choosing one. The greater this kind of reflective inner freedom a person has, the less reactive he or she will be, the more individuated he or she will become, and the more he or she will be able to handle the closeness of the HVR.

It is important that the therapist make clear to partners that disengagement and individuation do not mean permanent separation from the element. They can still merge with an element any time they wish. Now the merging will be under their executive control rather than under the control of their reactivity.

Following are examples of fusions of which the therapist can be aware and about which the therapist can raise awareness in the couple:

- Fusion with a Belief, Theory, School of Thought, or Philosophy of Life: In this case the person is attached to a theory or ideology to such extent that he or she is unable to step back, reflect on it, and critique it. The person does not hold it provisionally but rather with certainty. Disengaging and bracketing involves converting the theory into a hypothesis to be tested, thus making it an item for investigation, reflection, and evaluation. Without this bracketing, the fusion may contaminate any psychological growth work the person is doing.
- Fusion with a Person: Becoming individuated from one's parents (or parental surrogate) is probably the most important disengaging work partners can do. Without such disengagement, the partner will function as a Little Girl or Little Boy, subject to primitive pulls on his or her thoughts, feelings, and behavior. Even though the person may be geographically distant from the prototype figure, he or she will still hold the prototype in mind where it unconsciously influences life. Clues to this fusion include feeling disempowered, inadequate, confused, scared, guilty, ashamed, inferior, insecure, depressed, or dissociated.
- Fusion with an Inner Figure: Fusion with an inner figure leaves the person in the control of the figure. For example, a partner may be fused with a 4-year-old child inside who is making decisions without the person's awareness. Dialoguing with the figure will help the person become free.
- Fusion with the Inner Critic: Coerced and intimidated by this inner figure, the person may shape his or her life in accordance with its commands instead of living from the Natural Self.
- Fusion with the Reactive Self: Instead of following the guidance of the Natural Self, a partner may have found the Reactive Self so protective that he or she has fused with it. In order to grow through individuation, the partner will need to become free from the Reactive Self and choose loyalty to the Natural Self.

Using the Anthetic Rationality Sequence

Irrationality implies adopting magical principles instead of experientially tested ones and living by those principles even though they clearly lead to failure. Among irrational principles found in partners are these:

- I don't have to do any psychological work on myself in order to have a romantic HVR. All I need is love.
- If I obey my Inner Critic, I'll be happy.
- If I want to achieve my goals, I shouldn't talk about them to anyone.
- In choosing a life partner, I don't need to use criteria; I just need to ask myself if this is the real thing this time. That is, is it true love?
- I'm a Capricorn, and that accounts for my resistance and stubbornness.
- If a thing feels right in my gut, I'll do it, even though I wonder if it's really good for me.
- I don't like to think or talk about anything negative, because that just gives it more power.
- There's no such thing as the subconscious mind, so I don't have to wonder whether I'm acting from motives of which I'm unaware.
- I don't need to take feedback seriously, because I'm fully aware of everything that's going on in me.

In each of the above, and in other cases of irrational thinking, emotional seepage is functioning; that is, emotions seep into one's rationality and contaminate it. Seepage leads to unreflective decisions. For example, a person may marry someone impulsively and find out later that she is just like his or controlling mother or just like his or her remote father.

An important benefit of cultivating rationality is that it leads to psychological strength. That is, the Executive Self, guided by the Rational Self, helps in setting boundaries, avoiding gullibility, and making sound decisions. In order to achieve a well-trained Executive Self essential in optimal relating, Anthetic Relationship Therapy offers the following five steps of the Anthetic Rationality Sequence.

- Step One: For any given belief, convert absolute certainty to provisionality. This step requires that partners give up absolute certainty about everything they believe. This recommendation is based on the fact that some of a person's beliefs might actually be Cherished Dysfunctional Beliefs. The person will not know whether this is so if holding a certaintist position about them. Once put to the rationality testing process, some beliefs may be revealed as dysfunctional ones that are sabotaging the person's relationship.

  Each belief must be held provisionally, that is, converted to a hypothesis subject to revision in the light of possible new information. From this

standpoint, the person has the best chance of discovering which beliefs are valid and which are dysfunctional. Making beliefs provisional; that is, bracketing them temporarily and then examining them is the essential way to distinguish them. Once the person has converted certainties to provisionalities, the following tests may be applied to each belief.
- Step Two: Apply the stuffishness test. In this step, the therapist teaches the person to search for and process any psychological material that might be negatively influencing the belief, including not only wishful thinking but also any attachments to previously-held beliefs, especially those that have great value in buffering self-esteem.
- Step Three: Apply the invalidation test. In this step the therapist helps the person test each belief through a thoroughgoing search for evidence that it is wrong. This is achieved by carefully looking for exceptions that might invalidate the belief.
- Step Four: Apply the validation test. This step requires that the person find adequate and non-reactive reasons for holding the belief.
- Step Five: Be challengeable. Challengeability is the term for being open to being challenged and influenced. It involves welcoming challenges from others and considering them carefully instead of immediately rejecting them. Researching is an important part of this step.
- Step Six: Make the move to everyday confidence. Those beliefs that pass the above tests can then be moved into the category box labeled "Everyday Confidence." This means "something you are pretty sure of." Each such belief of which one is confident then is susceptible to bracketing and possible revision at any time. In essence, the person substitutes "Everyday Confidence" for "Absolute Certainty."

The above steps constitute Anthetic rationality. They are subject to modification or rejection, and more may be added. Following is an example from clinical practice:

Michael told the therapist he was certain his wife Marian had stopped loving him, and that he was sure she was planning to file for divorce. She had left him and was now living with her mother. As the therapist worked with Michael, he began with Step 1. He asked Michael to convert his certainty into a provisionality, that is, change it into a hypothesis to be tested. He did so.

In Step 2, they explored whether Michael's reactivity was affecting his belief. What emerged was an Inner Critic message predicting disaster and engendering magnified fear in Michael. Michael was able to factor out this item by challenging consisting of, "What do you know, Inner Critic? You're always telling me I'm so defective that nobody would ever love me."

In Step 3, Michael tested his belief by looking for contradictory evidence. He came up with the following, "She didn't say 'I want a divorce.' Nor did she say 'I don't love you anymore.'"

At the same time, the couple had been having ferocious arguments in which Marian had been complaining to Michael that he kept trying to micromanage her life, telling her that everything she was doing was wrong. Each morning, Michael had been leaving a list of things for Marian to do. Marian had finally rebelled against his attempts to control her.

With the therapist's help, Michael then formed a new hypothesis: "Maybe she isn't planning a divorce but is simply taking action to get away from my attempts to micromanage her behavior." This hypothesis proved to be the case.

Michael worked on the micromanaging impulses prescribed by his Inner Critic and ultimately became more easygoing. When this happened, Marian moved back home. The marriage prospered and began moving toward a high-voltage state.

Note that cultivating rationality does not mean giving up emotionality. The person still retains being in touch with his or her feelings and can still act on them. The principle of rationality holds that even though the decisions partners make may be based on emotion, they are best when evaluated by reason. Reason has the final say.

Chapter 7

Nine Skills to Empower the Self for Optimal Relating

The HVR model is a skills-based approach. In equipping couples who aspire to optimal relating, the therapist's task involves teaching the skills that make such relating possible. These skills are best seen in groups of the three foundations mentioned previously which have been carefully designed to equip couples with the best possible preparation for creating an HVR.

Foundation 1 skills comprise the basic guidelines: the concepts, values, and principles presented in Chapters 1 through 5. The therapist weaves these guidelines into the initial sessions and will continue to use them to inform the therapeutic process as it unfolds.

Foundation 2 skills are the intrapersonal skills for doing psychological work on oneself. The therapist will need to teach these *intra* skills (Chapters 3, 4, 6, and 7) before moving on to Foundation 3.

Foundation 3 skills are necessary for high-voltage communicating. These are the *inter* skills; those for interpersonal interactions (Chapters 8, 9, and 10).

The present chapter offers intrapersonal skills for partners' psychological work on themselves. If, for some reason, a partner finds it difficult to work at one of the Foundation 2 or 3 level (*intra* or *inter*), the therapist will need to guide the person back one level to focus on further work at the previous level. For example, were a partner to have difficulty at the *inter* level, the therapist may revert to addressing *intrapersonal* skills in order to dismantle any psychological blocks to using the interpersonal skills. If working at the *intra* level is difficult, the therapist may once again cover the basic guidelines of Foundation 1 to ensure the partner understands and accepts the guidelines. Finally, difficulty with basic guidelines indicates that a partner may need more intensive individual therapy in order to address psychological blocks and to build the executive self-strength to tolerate the voltage.

While the two primary Foundation 2 intrapersonal skills consist of Inner Critic work as well as Inner Figure work (presented in Chapters 3 and 4), additional intrapersonal skills are also needed to equip partners for optimal relating. Following are nine Foundation 2 intrapersonal skills necessary to support high-voltage relating.

Skill 1: Recovering from Self-Centeredness

Achievement of the HVR is predicated on partners' ability to engage and empathize with each other. This observation is supported by research showing that greater empathic ability is associated with greater marital satisfaction (Ickes, 1997; Geoff, Fletcher, & Lange, 1997). Frequently partners present with difficulty in empathizing with each other, a primary reason being self-centeredness.

An essential distinction must be made here, as partners often complain that the other is selfish. However, when questioned about the partner's behavior that led to this attribution, what the complainant describes is actually an example of self-centeredness. Selfishness is an excessive concern with the satisfaction of one's own needs over those of another. Although it may co-exist with empathy, selfishness is an absence of mutuality. The selfish person can perceive another person clearly but has consciously decided to hang on to everything he or she has, not to give anything. Self-centeredness, on the other hand, refers to an inability to perceive the other person clearly. When asked for something, a self-centered person may respond with help and even may be generous with time or possessions, but will have lacunae in perceiving the other person's feelings, wants, and needs. Self-centeredness at its core is a failure of empathy. The self-centered person is unable to truly be interested in other people, to give them "space" in their minds and to see them as separate individuals with their own needs, wishes, feelings, and interests.

In its clinical manifestation, self-centeredness appears as narcissism. Yet, even at sub-clinical levels, self-centeredness presents a barrier to achieving closeness. From a psychodynamic perspective, whether clinical or sub-clinical, self-centeredness is driven by both a history of failed attachment needs gratification along with Inner Critic injunctions to be perfect. Because empathizing with one's partner requires an ability to confront and contain the partner's painful or unhappy feelings, the self-centered person whose Inner Critic is powerful is vulnerable to decompensating in the face of feedback which disconfirms his or her self-image as a perfect person (Elliott, J., 1992a; Elliott, J., & Elliott, K., 2000). Maintaining emotional distance through a subconscious strategy of self-centeredness defends the person from anxiety that would be triggered were he or she to take into account the reality of the other person.

Strategies for maintaining a self-centered position in relationships comprise a number of communication patterns that include dominating a conversation. Being restricted to the role of listener often triggers feelings of humiliation secondary to Inner Critic messages that to listen to another means that the listener is inferior in status. For example, in a couple session, Ty asked Corinne not to interrupt so frequently. Her sarcastic response was then "Can I talk *now*?" repeated over and over. As the therapist helped Corinne describe her feelings, she indicated feelings of anxiety when in the role of listener.

In another case, Al and his wife Karen, just returning to therapy from a vacation trip by car from San Francisco down the coast to Los Angeles, described their interaction. About an hour into the drive, Al said, "I don't feel so good. I may not be the world's best vacation companion."

Karen's response was, "Oh, no! You're going to ruin my vacation!"

"Hey!" said Al. "What about me? You're just thinking about yourself!"

Karen realized the truth of his words immediately. "Guess I've got some self-centeredness to work on," she said.

The therapist then focused therapeutic work on helping Karen gain empathy skills.

A third case illustrates the broadcasting style of conversation indicative of self-centeredness. Peg and her partner Suzanne sought counseling for ongoing difficulties in their relationship. Peg began, "Suzanne, it's very painful when we talk, because you don't see me, and I can't get a word in edgewise. And you keep interrupting me whenever I try." Suzanne admitted feeling hurt at this feedback. As the session proceeded, she remained defensive about the feedback. Because Suzanne was unable to emotionally tolerate the Foundation 3 interpersonal process, the therapist guided her into Foundation 2 intrapersonal work, focusing on Inner Figure work and Inner Critic challenging.

A final example of communication strategies that evidence self-centeredness is free association. Payton, a married man in individual therapy, lamented, "I tell my wife Caitlin something, and she never responds to what I say. She just responds with whatever she is thinking or feeling that has nothing to do with what I said." The therapist suggested Payton bring Caitlin for a couple session, which he did. As the session progressed, realization dawned that Caitlin's free association was a defense against Inner Critic shoulds to be a perfect wife. After she learned to challenge her Inner Critic, she was able to welcome and process her husband's conversational overtures, including disconfirmatory feedback. They were both delighted with this new way of communicating.

In helping a couple to recover from self-centeredness, the therapist must address five tasks. First, because the self-centered person is unaware of his or her self-centeredness, the therapist must assist in converting this defensive pattern from an ego-syntonic perspective that holds the self-centered behavior as normal to an ego-dystonic one, that is, seeing the self-centeredness as reactive material from which to become free. Once the individual gains such understanding, the therapist then facilitates the person making a Request for Targeted Feedback (Chapter 9) of the partner: "Tell me whenever you see me being self-centered, because I want to get free from it."

Second, the therapist must empower the person with processing skills for benefiting from targeted feedback (Chapter 5). In the third task, the person who struggles with self-centeredness learns to work on his or her impatience, so as to tolerate other people's speaking (Chapter 6). The fourth task involves learning to be interested in other people, to ask them Interested Questions (Chapter 8). In the fifth task, the person learns the skill of empathizing (Chapter 10).

While these tasks can be quite difficult for the person with self-centeredness to undertake, he or she can usually make progress by providing positive reinforcement in the form of praise and approval from the partner and therapist when doing one of the tasks.

Skill 2: Accessing Neediness

Empirical research supports that humans are born needy for reliable, frequent, positive, and loving interactions (Baumeister & Leary, 1995; Bowlby, 1988). Not only are love and closeness essential for both physical and mental health, but they also are fundamental for optimal functioning and for happiness (Myers & Diener, 1995; Ryff, 1989). Further, neurophysiology research has shown the need for love in humans to be a physiologically powerful motivation state involving complex neurological interactions.

Such research reveals that the drive for romantic love is a function of reward and goal representation regions of the brain (Aron, Fisher, Mashek, Strong, Haifang, & Brown, 2005).

Despite this innate need for security in love that continues throughout the lifespan (Bowlby, 1988), fulfillment of this drive is frequently thwarted by attachment wounds in the parent-child bond (Collins & Read, 1990; Feeney & Noller, 1990; Hazan & Shaver, 1987; Levy, Blatt, & Shaver, 1998; Rothbard & Shaver, 1994). Such wounds have continuing impact on thoughts, feelings, attitudes, and behavior in adult romantic relationships (see Feeney, J.A., 1999 for a review of these findings).

The pain of attachment wounds is so great that children cope with it by adopting one of the four Anthetic Polar personality styles (Chapter 3). Those who function from a Tender and/or Dependent style will still be in touch with their emotional neediness. On the other hand, those who cope through a Tough or Self-Sufficient style submerge neediness, as commanded by their

Inner Critics, concluding that they do not have the right to be needy or in emotional pain. In therapy, when the topic of emotional neediness emerges, the Tough or Self-Sufficient person will typically evidence their aversion to neediness by grimacing.

In clinical research, the ability to access neediness is essential for an HVR. When emotional neediness is submerged, the therapist may facilitate freedom by assisting the person with releasing statements to take back the right to be needy. As dysfunctional beliefs consisting of shoulds stored in the person's Inner Critic become conscious, and the person becomes skilled in challenging them, the power of attachment wounds to cause emotional pain reduces, as does their negative impact on intimate relationships.

Skill 3: Recovering from Counter-Humiliation

Humilophobia is the Anthetic term for fear of feeling humiliated. Each polar type experiences feelings of humiliation when touching, even momentarily, the opposite pole's features. Many couple problems are caused by counter-humiliation programs, which develop in order to curtail the pain of humiliation triggered when intimate relations evoke opposite pole features. Examples of counter-humiliation follow:

- Humiliation for following directions: In teaching couples the interpersonal skill, for example, requesting, the therapist guides partners to "Say the requesting sequence word for word. Don't improvise at this point." Some partners disregard these directions and say whatever feels natural. When the therapist gently corrects the partner, the person is often surprised to learn that they had been doing the skill incorrectly and makes statements such as the following: "I didn't want to parrot you"; "I didn't want to be a carbon copy of you"; and "I didn't want to knuckle under to you." Upon further inquiry, the person explained that parroting, carbon-copying, and knuckling under would make them look weak, and that would be humiliating. Inner Critic work helped them identify these beliefs as dysfunctional ones that presented blocks to learning skills for closeness. This recognition is important for therapists, who may incorrectly view the person's defensive behavior as obstinance rather than as a counter-humiliation program that is driving the behavior. In addition, occasionally a person will attempt to justify noncompliance by saying, "I've spent years being controlled by other people, and now I'm going to do what I want to do." In this case, reactivity masquerades as assertiveness. Reactive assertiveness may, however, prevent the person from engaging in the learning necessary to create optimal high-voltage relating. The distinguishing clue to reactivity is this: If the person lacks *psychological flexibility*, he or she will be unable to disrupt automatic behavior and will not have the option to either be assertive or submissive when either would enhance functioning and relating optimally. Such ability to be psychologically flexible rests on partners choosing to prioritize the values of inner freedom, emotional closeness, and flexibility over other values, including assertiveness.

- Humiliation about expressing love: Counter-humiliation programs often prevent people from complying with requests from their partners for love and affection. Clinical evidence reveals such difficulty as having its source in past learning from personal experiences and from the culture. In the case of Jed, this past learning was connected to an incident in grade school. "In the third grade," he revealed, "I wrote a little love poem to a girl I had a crush on. The teacher found it and read it to the class. Everybody laughed. I decided never to be mushy again." From that moment forward anti-mushiness became a counter-humiliation strategy for him. Without the ability to express love and affection, his attempts at having a HVR were unsuccessful: partners who adopt a low-voltage style of relating often have great difficulty expressing love and say, "Don't push me. I can't do it on demand. I'll do it when I'm ready." Their partners frequently become frustrated, because becoming ready does not happen. In contrast, partners who adopt an HVR style can usually express love on demand. Their ability to do so is based on freedom from Inner Critic condemnation of loving expressiveness along with flexibility to be both loving and assertive.
- Uncoolness as humiliation: Avoidance of being seen as "not cool" is a counter-humiliation program with roots primarily in junior high and high school. Consider the case of Gayla, whose husband requested she use her turn signal while driving. She readily admitted in therapy that she was puzzled by this inability to comply with a request that seemed quite easy to do. Exploration of the roots of her non-compliance revealed that in high school she was a member of a clique that was characterized by a "don't give a damn about anything" culture. She stated, "I was a cheerleader, a popular girl. You were supposed to be cool. Or you were humiliated." When she realized that she was still living her life as though performing for her high school friends, she was able to declare a new decision to live as the loving partner to which she aspired rather than as a teen girl seeking acceptance at all costs from her peers. She was then free to use her turn signal as requested by her husband. Her case illustrates how valuing being cool builds walls between people that will prevent the HVR from being created.
- Knuckling under as humiliation: As mentioned previously, for some people, complying with a request may be seen through a filter that converts

it into opprobrious "knuckling under." This is especially correlated with those who function from a rigid Tough or Self-Sufficient position.

For example, when Jerome heard Debbie request that he leave the lights on in the downstairs rooms in the house, even though she was using only one room, he bristled. "It's ridiculous," he said. "A waste of money! Why should I do what she wants?" he asked the therapist. "I'm definitely not going to be an obedient little wimp." As the therapist explored the roots of this position with him, he revealed that he was influenced by learning he had heard in his childhood from his father: "Don't let a woman get you under her thumb." This learning had become a firmly held dysfunctional belief. In counseling, the therapist taught Jerome to disengage from the early learning filter and to make a decision to value inner freedom along with caring. At the therapist's suggestion, he gained a different perspective, seeing his reaction to Debbie as reactivity; specifically, an Inner Critic issue blocking him from complying with an Easy to Do Request requisite to a HVR (Chapter 9).

"Okay," he told the therapist. "I suppose I need to make a releasing statement." The therapist replied yes and asked if he could formulate one.

Jerome thought for a while then stated, "Oh, no! I can't believe it! I can't say it."

The therapist asked, "Are you thinking the challenge to your Inner Critic is, 'I have the right to let a woman get me under her thumb? I have the right to be what my Inner Critic calls an obedient wimp?'"

When Jerome said yes, the therapist directed him in preliminary Anthetic Dialogue with his prototype; that is, his father imagined as sitting in the empty chair. He realized that his belief was indeed a highly valued dysfunctional belief. The father's message led to Jerome's characterizing compliance with any request from a woman as weakness, which he called "wimpiness." Jerome reflected, "I think this is why Debbie and I have so many arguments. Okay. I have the right to knuckle under to a woman, and I have the right to be a hen-pecked wimp." These words were accompanied by a grimace. Such facial gestures are indicative that the releasing statement contained material about a topic so highly charged with negative emotion that it produced somatic manifestations. The therapist provided Jerome perspective, "Of course, this is not really about knuckling under or being a wimp. Those are the terms your Inner Critic uses to constrict your life by pejoritizing the situation." The dynamics of Jerome's block consisted of a symbolic overlay, in which, to a neutral request, he added symbolic meaning from dysfunctional learning.

- Being one down as humiliation: Because being one down is felt as humiliation, partners will strive at all costs to be one up. Being one down may be associated with following directions, being instructed by someone, asking for advice, and losing the game of conversational competition, and (as in the case of Jerome above) complying with a request. When therapists refer to a power struggle between partners, what they usually are referring to can now be seen as a clash of counter-humiliation programs. The struggle occurs in a subconscious attempt to avoid the humiliation of losing the buffer of winning or being one up.

- Connecting as humiliation: When partners have difficulty connecting in conversations, counter-humiliation is operating. To respond directly to a question, for example, might not only be a humiliating experience in itself because of its symbolic overlay (e.g., knuckling under), it might also mean disclosing a humiliating situation (e.g., exhibiting ignorance by saying, "I don't know the answer to that question").
- Asking questions as humiliation: Counter-humiliation strategies are evident when a person has difficulty asking questions. Examples include asking for directions in a strange town and asking for definitions of terms in class. Therefore, people pretend to knowledge they do not possess, hoping no one will notice. In turn, others, even when they do notice, do not challenge the person who pretends to knowledge, partially out of politeness. Other reasons include anticipatory empathy of the humiliation the person would feel at exposure of his or her ignorance as well as perception of the pretense as a form of touchiness indicative of fragility. The outcome of this dynamic is distance in the relationship. Over time this pattern will produce a LVR.
- Being tested and evaluated as humiliation: One important feature of high-voltage relating involves asking for feedback on one's progress in mastering the skills and in producing closeness. A partner who views being tested or evaluated as humiliating will be unable to tolerate engaging in these valuable activities. For the partner who experiences humiliation, the structure is often a reliance on a compensatory buffer (e.g., pride in being perfect) for self-esteem. Were the partner to hear that he or she was not doing well at mastering one of the skills, the buffer would collapse, exposing the person to Inner Critic emotional punishments, particularly shame. If the therapist can engage the partner in Foundation 1 work by assisting the partner in making a value shift from pride to optimal high voltage relating, counter-humiliation will no longer be a driving factor. Instead, the partner can learn to embrace any humiliation that might be triggered, whereupon he or she can challenge the Inner Critic to reduce the pain of the humiliation.

In order to reverse counter-humiliation programs, likely the most important obstacle to having an HVR, partners must be able to identify and dismantle the programs, thus enabling them to tolerate learning the skills necessary for optimal relating. In other words, couple communication problems are more complex than merely lacking surface skills. If a partner is stonewalling or withdrawn, it is now clear that stubbornness or hard-heartedness are not the problem, but rather is an underlying fear of humiliation. Were the person to open up emotionally, powerful self-condemnatory forces would be unleashed. Therefore to neutralize these forces, partners must acquire proficiency in Inner Critic challenging before interpersonal skills of openness can be learned. Anthetic Relationship Therapy guides couples in a three step process for dismantling counter-humiliation programs:

1. First, partners must welcome feelings of humiliation, even going out of their way to experience them, and then embrace them. This step can be done once partners see the role the Inner Critic plays in producing counter-humiliation programs.
2. Second, partners must do Anthetic Inner Critic work to reduce or eliminate the power of the feelings of humiliation.
3. Third, partners must begin to work toward giving up their need to protect their cherished self-image, that is, buffered self-image, from disconfirmatory feedback. This step is possible once partners understand and choose the value of inner freedom, recognizing its importance in not only feeling self-accepting but also in tolerating and enjoying closeness.

Skill 4: Anthetic Self-Analysis and Clue Work

In order to achieve psychological growth, a primary value in optimal relating, partners must gain the ability to engage in self-analysis. The Anthetic Relationship Therapy term, Anthetic Self-Analysis, refers to the ability to explore one's subconscious machinery that drives a thought, feeling, attitude, or behavior. At the heart of this exploration is curiosity about oneself, along with the capacity to ask "Why?" questions. Two kinds of analysis can be employed: horizontal and vertical.

Horizontal analysis involves asking oneself whether a problem appears in a number of areas and with a number of people. For example, if a person has difficulty being assertive, does that happen only with the person's partner or also with one's boss, employees, and teachers?

Vertical analysis goes deeper into subconscious motivations. The general form of one statement a person can use to practice this skill is, "I wonder why I did that." A variation of the skill is, "I wonder what that was about." A version of this skill useful in exploring Inner Figure structures is, "Who are you?" asked in order to evoke Inner Figure dialogue. These questions are meant as an opening to inner material; a form of wonderment that kindles a meditation on subconscious motivation. In keeping with anthetic relationship

Therapy philosophy, they provide clients with portable skills that they may use outside the therapy session and for the rest of their lives.

As the therapist and client engage in the anthetic self-analysis process, certain clues will begin to emerge. A clue is an element in one's conscious mind that, if pursued at successively deeper levels, will lead to the discovery of what has been driving one's reactive behavior and limiting one's inner freedom. Common clues include puzzling behavior, thoughts, feelings, mistakes, and occasions of procrastination and forgetfulness. Clue Work will exhibit how the person has been limiting his or her inner freedom.

An important caution in clue work is that the therapist and client must not occlude the clue by prematurely correcting any mistake. Clue-occlusion will prevent one from gleaning the message of the clue. The person may achieve a more polished self-presentation via shaping and constricting the self but will miss the opportunity for achieving greater inner freedom. The following clinical example illustrates this possible error:

ROXANNE: "I really should follow the rules."

THERAPIST: "Don't say 'should.' Convert the should into a want."

ROXANNE: "Oh, okay. I *want* to follow the rules."

Roxanne's supposed mistake has now been corrected; however, she has learned nothing about inner freedom. Instead, she has learned to say something in a supposed right way, thus achieving a polished performance. Change that has occurred is of a cosmetic nature, not one that increases inner freedom from subconscious material.

Had Roxanne pursued the goal of inner freedom, she would have challenged her Inner Critic, then used the should as a clue to her general constrictedness through some influence from the past. She might then have made the following statement: "I have the right to say 'should' any time I want."

Following is a list of questions the therapist and client may ask that can lead to additional ways to do Clue Work:

- "Was my Inner Critic involved? If so, what was the should?"
- "What other inner figures are blocking me? My Little Boy? My Little Girl?"
- "Is my pride getting in the way?"
- "Is one of my prototype inner figures blocking me? Loyalty to Mom or Dad? Or someone else?"
- "Do I have the right values for optimal functioning? Inner freedom? Pleasure instead of revenge? Being a grownup?"
- "Might my problem be caused by a drive for revenge?"

- In addition, the client can learn the following "Why?" questions about a number of items. For example:
- "I wonder why I didn't apply for that job I really wanted."
- "I wonder why I feel so trapped in this relationship."
- "I wonder why I seem so driven to control the details of my partner's life."
- "I wonder why I have so much trouble being assertive."
- "I wonder why I am so touchy when I get feedback."
- "I wonder why I have to win every argument I have at all costs, by fair means or foul."
- "I wonder why I keep picking partners who are bad for me,"

  As these Clue Work questions are explored, the therapist can guide the person is avoiding common errors that prevent profiting by such Clue Work:
- Giving easy excuse answers. For example, saying "I don't talk to my wife about serious issues because there just isn't enough time." Clue work would involve looking for reasons the person chooses not to.
- Giving terminal-trait answers. For example, saying, "I didn't apply for the job because I'm lazy"; "Well, who wouldn't be touchy if she or he got negative feedback"; "I can't talk about my feelings because I'm a private person"; "Who wouldn't be angry if someone humiliated him?" or "I can't be assertive because I'm too insecure." Such answers are simply redescriptions of the problem and do not add explanations in terms of underlying dynamics.
- Avoiding looking for the payoff involved in having the problem. The therapist can offer the following incomplete sentence to counter this problem: "I really appreciate having this problem, because it gives me ________." One clinical example occurred with a partner who had great difficulty in pursuing her spouse for connection, yet felt lonely and isolated. As the therapist guided her in searching for a possible payoff she found, "I really want loneliness and isolation, because then I'll send a message to Mom and Dad about how bad their training of me was."
- Giving quick diagnostic answers. An example of this block is, "I can't change my passive behavior, because I'm a masochist." Instead, the person can be assisted in looking deeper, for example, looking for connections to the Inner Critic, uncovering shoulds, challenging them. Further Clue Work may reveal that there are multiple reasons for the difficulty.

A case example of Clue Work in Anthetic Relationship Therapy involves Clarice. Clarice and her husband Nick sought therapy for Clarice's rage at Nick. Clarice admitted to feeling chagrin that her rage flared up every three or four days and always at seemingly unimportant issues. In doing an analysis her first step was to discard superficial answers, "Because it's that time of the month"; "Because I just have a hot temper"; "Because he leaves his socks on the bedroom floor"; "Because I'm tired from all the work I have to do"; "Because this is just the battle of the sexes."

With the help of the therapist, she began a serious examination of her thoughts and feelings at a deeper level. She began exploring vertically.

"He's a man," she said, "and men are always oppressing women. He keeps criticizing me because I'm too emotional. He says I keep contradicting myself. But to me, I just feel confused when he questions me. I freeze."

As the session proceeded, Clarice gained valuable insight. First, she was replaying a scenario from her childhood, when she had a sadistic teacher. The teacher was relentless in his angry criticism, making each student stand up and recite until they had all achieved perfection. As a student, she responded by becoming flustered. Her mind was a blank.

As she opened herself to the meaning of her rage at Nick, she was surprised to discover that: (a) Her rage was usually triggered by ordinary questions from Nick, such as "How were the kids today?" (b) Although she knew perfectly well how the kids were, she gave a confused and contradictory answer, just as she had in school, (c) She realized her confused answer was an attempt at revenge on Nick. She felt disempowered but knew the one thing he hated was her ignorance. So she inflicted that ignorance on him just to make him feel angry. Clarice's husband was a stand-in for her teacher. She was gaining symbolic revenge on her teacher. This analysis revealed that emotional pain from her past had been intruding in her marriage.

In therapy, she did Anthetic Dialogue work with her teacher imagined as occupying an empty chair. Her rage, directed now at the right person who was the source of her pain, diminished somewhat, but there seemed to be some other mechanism that was still driving it. As she continued in therapy she saw that she had been fusing with a Spiteful Little Girl inner figure. When she was able to identify this figure and orchestrate it, the rage at her husband disappeared.

The Anthetic Relationship Therapy term for the unfolding process in which Clarice engaged is called a linking process; connecting the present with dysfunctional past learnings (the prototypes), so those learnings can be unlearned and replaced with new and more effectual learning.

Skill 5: Recognizing and Resisting Pulls

Although Clarice was able through Self-Analysis and Clue Work to identify the structure of her reactive rage, an additional step was needed to equip her to become free from habitual act-outs of that structure. The Spiteful Little Girl was "put on the shelf." However, Clarice still felt an impulse from the inner figure to let it play its part in her life. The therapist offered her the Anthetic Relationship Therapy intervention of *Pull Reports.* This technique involves recognizing, reporting, resisting, and analyzing dysfunctional impulses (or pulls). She spotted and reported the pull by saying "I feel a pull from my Spiteful Little Girl." Next she used Anthetic Rationality to evaluate the pull: "Is this beneficial to my growth? Or my marriage? Or is it harmful?" Then she used Anthetic Dialogue to tell the Spiteful Little Girl, "I'm not going to let you wreck my marriage." Finally, she said, "I choose magnanimity over spiteful rage." In addition, she reported the pull by saying, "I feel a pull to be spiteful, but I'm not going to go there."

This process required a value shift. Her new non-rueful behavior now grew naturally from her Loving Self. No willpower was needed. She could be alert to feeling the pull again, whereupon, she could again do the challenging and reporting. Pull work consists of the following steps:

1. Identify the pull and report it.
2. If it is dysfunctional, challenge it by saying "I'm not going to go there."
3. Analyze the pull. Use methods presented in the Self-Analysis and Clue Work section.
4. Make a value shift. Surrender loyalty to the value embedded in the pull, and substitute a more functional value.
5. Make a targeted feedback request. Ask the partner, "Let me know every time you see me acting out the pull."

Skill 6: Developing Affect Tolerance

An affect is a subjective feeling or emotion, together with whatever physiological responses are also present. Affect tolerance is the ability to carry out the processes of rational thinking, sound decision-making, and responsible behavior even though one is flooded with feelings. It includes not automatically giving in to whatever pressures one feels. The net result is that partners live a psychologically principled life rather than an impulse-directed life.

Affect tolerance includes the ability to bear disappointment, emotional pain, anxiety, and loneliness without being overwhelmed. It involves the ability to confront and accept feelings of sexuality, hostility, passivity, and aggression. Employing affect tolerance entails the skill to confront the Inner Critic directly in order to target challenges accurately. It also means the capability to resist enmeshment and other fusions, as well as to withstand emotional pressures one feels from other people. Most important, it means being able to handle feelings of humiliation and to report dysfunctional pulls instead of capitulating to them.

The skill of affect tolerance is involved in almost every task presented in this book. Basically, it is a form of impulse control, as well as a prerequisite for individuation. It is essential for creating a successful HVR.

In order to achieve proficiency in affect tolerance, some clients are able to do so through simple desensitization as they experience more and more strong affects and give themselves the self-soothing message, "Feelings are not facts. They are just feelings" (Low, 1950). Additionally, the client may combine this assertion with the Anthetic method of Inner Critic challenging, "Just because I experience strong feelings doesn't mean I have to do a thing." Undergirding these skills, the client can make use of slowing down and relaxing, as well as biofeedback strategies for reducing diffuse physiological arousal (Gottman, 1999).

However, when these strategies fail, the therapist and client may use the Anthetic Relationship Therapy protocol for *Anxiety Containment.* When couples become extremely reactive in session, the therapist can become reactive also; feeling an impulse to yell at the clients or be punitive by saying, "I can't help you—you should just divorce." The Anthetic psychodynamic explanation for this is twofold: First, the client's reactivity is seen as an acted out lament. Second, the therapist's reactivity is understood as anxiety triggered by the client's acted out reactivity. Following is the Anthetic therapeutic intervention for Anxiety Containment:

Step 1: The therapist labels his or her internal state, "This is just anxiety."
Step 2: The therapist contains the emotions in the session using labeling and empathy both to her self or himself and to clients.
Step 3: The therapist inwardly reflects, "This client is lamenting a core wound and needs empathy. I want to empathize."
Step 4: To the client, the therapist (not necessarily in this order):
  a. Offers the Anthetic Sacrament, "I'm so sorry you. . . ."
  b. Asks, "Can you tell me more about that?"
  c. Offers an empathic double.
  d. Teaches concepts to equip the client to understand and disengage from anxiety; primarily "the mine field metaphor," the lament, and the Anthetic Sacrament (given to oneself and to one's partner) (Chapter 9).

Skill 7: Developing Impulse Control: Learning to Focus

In order to disrupt spontaneous machinelike behavior, the individual must learn to separate impulses from actions. The therapist teaches the client to do this through the *Just* Because challenge, "Just because I have an impulse doesn't mean I have to act it out." This is a releasing statement, addressed to the Inner Critic, who may have been supplying the message that act-outs are normal and acceptable (Elliott, J., 1991). A person who has accepted this perspective may as a result behave from a Regressed Child level rather than an adult level. Unable to engage in focused thinking, they are unable to speak in a focused way. Speaking impulsively, without thinking first, can result in splattering, that is, not addressing the topic but instead talking disconnectedly by giving free associations to the topic. This associational manner of speaking is produced by a Child inner figure who wants to avoid humiliation by offering a series of smokescreens, hoping no one will notice. It is a defensive maneuver to avoid Inner Critic pain. The result of this type of functioning will prevent high-voltage relating, as the ability to focus and control one's behavior at the direction of one's Executive Self is an important high-voltage skill. In order to help a person become free of impulsive, unfocused responding, the therapist must first teach Inner Critic challenging, thus freeing the person from the defensive structure created to avoid Inner Critic emotional punishment.

Skill 8: Cultivating Psychological Flexibility

A primary block to high-voltage relating occurs when partners are either disengaged from one another in a crystallized way or are merged with one another in a crystallized way. In Anthetic Therapy the term *detachment* is used to refer to this form of rigid disengagement and is akin to what Ickes, Hutchison, and Mashek (2004) labeled individuated aloofness. The term fusion is used in Anthetic Therapy to refer to rigid merging, similar to the state called deindividuated merging by Ickes, et al. Either states will prevent the achievement of a successful HVR.

What is needed instead is anthetic orthogonal flexibility, in which partners are free from fusions and rigid positions. Each functions from provisionality, the ability to disengage or to merge as he or she freely chooses. Each functions essentially as a free spirit, capable of what Ickes, et al., refer to as individuated interdependence, where the sense of self and the sense of other-in-relationship are both high. Anthetic Relationship Therapy uniquely adds the concept of flexibility, in which free choice is activated, made possible by freedom from the Inner Critic, inner figures, and prototype influences.

Skill 9: Working toward Individuation

In order to function in a provisional manner, each partner must work toward individuation. The term implies the ability to differentiate from one's family of origin, from one's partner, and from others toward whom one feels the pull of permanent fusion. In addition, the term refers to disengaging from any ideology or philosophical system and bracketing it so one can begin from an equiprimordial position. Further, individuation includes (through a process of self-exploration) having progressively increasing access to all the potentials that exist in one's psyche (Jung, 1956). As partners gain freedom to deploy any of those potentials, each person becomes more and more an individual rather than a machinelike simulacrum. One gradually surrenders a stultifying herd mentality, becoming what Heidegger (1962) termed *eigentlich* (one's own self) and what Sartre (1956) called living *pour soi* (for yourself), no longer living as a material object, *en soi* (in itself).

As the individuation process continues, the person no longer remains trapped by a driven over-concern with what other people think of him or her and thus is less addicted to others' approval. In this state, the person may live from the natural self instead of the reactive self, disengaging increasingly from shoulds imposed by the Inner Critic. Moreover, the individual no longer rigidly functions from only one polar type, but instead can freely choose any of them. Most important, for the process of helping couples in therapy, Anthetic orthogonal individuation is the crucial process that serves as the foundation for learning each of the skills for high-voltage relating. Of course, such individuation is an ongoing life process.

Chapter 8

Creating Connection

The Interpersonal High-Voltage Communication Skills

A deep sense of emotional closeness is a core foundation for not only mental health but also for optimal functioning (Bowlby, 1988; Epstein, 1994; Collins & Feeney, 2000). Research finds that in order to create the relationship climate of soothing and negotiating conducive to optimality, that is, a safe haven for self-disclosure, the couple's style of *start-up* is essential. In fact, John Gottman's now classic findings indicate that the first minute of couple communication is useful in predicting divorce or stability (Gottman, 1999). Harsh start-ups in which partners escalated into negative affect were associated with marital instability and divorce. Softened start-ups evidenced by expressions of good will were indicative of marital health. Anthetic Relationship Therapy holds that for optimal HVRs, the couple needs skills for creating connection that not only is characterized by emotional closeness evoked by the therapist while in session but also sustainable by the couple in everyday conversations. Such skills are readily teachable to partners beginning with the first session of therapy.

Identifying the Lament

As partners present in therapy, their first communications are most often indicative of the pain each is experiencing. Harsh start-ups marked by complaints, criticism, and tearful accusations, along with stonewalling exhibited by withdrawal and silence are all indicators that the partners are in deep emotional pain but lack the skill to speak of it effectively. Typically, unskilled partners fail to identify these expressions of pain with resultant escalation of affective expression (flooding) or movement into deeper stonewalling noted by researchers (Gottman, 1999). In Anthetic Relationship Therapy, the therapist conceptualizes all such expressions of emotional pain and labels each as a lament. This conceptualization guides the therapist in assessing the couple for expressions of emotional pain. As the therapist identifies the partner's laments, he or she offers this concept to the couple. Couples typically respond with an expressed sense of understanding and of being understood, as was demonstrated in the following session with Joan and Paul.

In their first session, Joan and Paul, both in their second marriage, reported they had been engaging in cyclic volatile arguments occurring every two weeks. During the arguments and again in the session, Joan complained, "You never listen to me, Paul! I try and try to tell you my hurt feelings and you just won't listen. I feel like I'm going crazy!" Joan noted that the arguments often resulted in her pleading with him through tears. Joan said, "I feel like I used to feel with my mother. I'd go to her in some distress and she'd say, 'You're just crazy!' I ended up feeling like maybe I *was* crazy!"

Paul, in turn, noted that during their arguments, he would begin feeling more and more anxious. He told Joan, "Nothing I do is ever enough. I've changed my clothes for you; I've bought you the car you wanted. Now you want something else. Nothing is ever, ever enough! I've had it!" Paul reported that when these arguments occurred at home, he would finally retreat to his home office or would leave the home. He reported with some chagrin even having at times yelled at Joan, "Get out!"

The therapist responded to this description of the structure of their arguments by offering the concept of the lament. "I want to give you a term that I think will help you understand what is happening between you. It's the concept of the lament." A brief psychoeducational moment explained further. "A lament is a cry of pain. You know how a person may wake up with a backache and cry out, 'Aargh!' That is a lament about physical pain. Likewise, when we feel emotional pain, we cry out too. It can be expressed in a number of ways: complaints, tears, anger, and even silence. What I have heard each of you say are expressions of your emotional pain to each other—your laments. Does that make sense?"

Both Joan and Paul responded in a manner that evidenced understanding. Joan said, "That really fits. I am in pain each time I tell Paul he isn't listening to me. I'm usually in tears." In turn Paul reflected, "I hadn't thought of it like that, but it does make sense. I try so hard to please Joan. I just want her to be happy. But when it seems that nothing I do is enough, it hurts. I know it comes out like anger, but underneath I really am hurt. It's exactly how I felt when my mother used to rely on me to help her raise my older disabled brother alone. No matter how much I knocked myself out, she always wanted something more from me."

The therapist, utilizing this moment of understanding, offered another concept which the couple could use to respond to each other's laments in a manner that deepens connection. As Paul had spoken last, she addressed

Joan, "Joan, did you realize that Paul's complaints and anger during your arguments were expressions of pain; were in fact, his lament?"

Joan responded, "No, I didn't, but I see it now."

The Anthetic Sacrament as Deep Empathy

As the couple encounters each other's pain in the light of the new concept of the lament, an important potential for connecting arises. Essential to closeness is the expression of empathy. The therapist probed further, "Do you feel some empathy for Paul as you listen to him now?"

Joan unhesitatingly replied, "Yes, I *do*."

The therapist then offered the anthetic relationship therapy skill termed the anthetic sacrament. "Would you say to Paul (if it's true), 'I'm so sorry you've felt with me at times like what you do isn't enough, because you deserve to feel seen and appreciated for all you do for me.'" The therapist amended, "I want to explain that this 'I'm sorry' is not an apology; it's more like the expression of heart-felt empathy we offer when we say to the bereaved at a funeral home, 'I'm so sorry for your loss.' It is not a message of responsibility; simply a deeply understanding expression of caring and love."

Joan then turned to Paul and said, quite tenderly, "I am so sorry that you've felt as though what you do is not enough. You *do* deserve to feel seen and appreciated for all you do for me." Then she spontaneously added, "And I want to say I know how hard it was for you as a child that your mother depended on you so much. And I really feel so sorry that sometimes what I say or ask feels like that childhood pain all over again." At that point, Paul's eyes began to overflow with tears, and he reached out to grab Joan's hand.

The therapist then asked Paul, "Paul do you feel some empathy for Joan's pain that she said occurs for her?"

Paul unhesitatingly responded, "Yes! I do."

At this point, the therapist asked Paul to turn to Joan and express his empathy using the words, "I'm so sorry you've felt not listened to by me."

Paul, still holding Joan's hand, offered, "I am so sorry you have felt I don't listen to you. And that it feels like the old pain from your Mom when she'd call you 'crazy.' You deserve to be listened to with respect."

As soon as Paul's words were spoken, Joan began to sob, and they both fell into each other's arms, weeping. As partners speak such words of empathy, the tone in the room becomes what Anthetic therapists characterize as a "sacred moment." The profundity of the reconciliation between previously conflictual partners is undeniable.

The Anthetic Sacrament provides a skill through which partners may reach a moment of completed empathic attunement. The closeness is achieved through what Ickes and colleagues (Ickes, 1997; Ickes & Simpson, 1997) have called *empathic accuracy* defined as the degree of accuracy partners are able to attain in response to shared feelings of the other. The therapist formalizes the process for the couple. "What you've just done is what is called in Anthetic Relationship Therapy, *The Anthetic Sacrament.* It's a communication in which pain is met with empathy. Because of the depth of connection, as you've just experienced, is so profound, we felt it had the weight of a sacred moment; a sacrament. It is a psychological sacrament, of course, not a religious one.

"When a couple experiences, as you have, those cycling arguments, they're bursting to speak their laments. Now that you are recognizing your own and each other's laments as cries of pain, you can begin the task of reconciling; becoming closer. For what is essential in reconciliation is that the person with the lament needs to receive deep empathy; to know their pain is seen and understood. You have just experienced it."

Joan and Paul both commented, "It certainly did feel like a sacred moment. Anthetic Sacrament: We like that."

The therapist then suggested to the couple that the Anthetic Sacrament is a skill they may use at home. The couple, as with each couple involved in Anthetic Relationship Therapy, was encouraged to begin to translate this skill to their communications at home. The therapist suggests to the couple that they can learn to identify laments communicated by their partner, beginning with the cyclic lament exhibited in this session. The therapist further explains that any complaint, angry comment, tears, or even withdrawal into silence can be seen as a lament, an expression of pain. Once the lament is recognized, the listening partner can offer the Anthetic Sacrament to the lamenting one. They are encouraged to become conscious and mindful of the process outside of the therapy session and to share with the therapist any opportunities that arose for practicing this skill.

Initiating a Conversation

Having learned to address pain of laments through the skill of the Anthetic Sacrament, the couple has become equipped to address stress and create a foundation for a safe haven. However, as Rook (1987) noted, individuals enter social relationships not just for support during times of stress but also for companionship and connection during non-stressful times. Partners seeking optimal relationships articulate this need by asking, "How do we relate now that we're not fighting?"

In LVRs, partners usually limit themselves to talking about themselves or surface topics. This conversational style lacks energy, intensity, and vitality. The low-voltage category compares to what ENRICH typology (Olson & Olson, 1999) classifies as devitalized couples, who have the lowest levels of intimacy and less capacity to deal with stressors. In contrast, high-voltage partners are comparable to what ENRICH classifies as vitalized couples, that is, the most intimate and skilled, their communications marked by emotional connection and flexibility to adapt to stress. Kouneski & Olson (2004) note that closeness within a couple is the best predictor of intimacy. In fact, couples in which both partners perceive a high level of closeness were twelve times more likely to present as vitalized.

One essential skill offered to couples in Anthetic Relationship Therapy is the start-up communication skill of *initiating conversations.* This skill consists of a partner exercising personal power by speaking first and declaring their thoughts, feelings, and intentions in a proactive manner. Examples of initiating include reporting feelings (e.g., "I'm feeling a bit awkward"); revealing a thought (e.g., "I'm thinking of our visit with your mother last week"); and statements of desires or intentions (e.g., "I want us to take a drive together today").

Couples may present two types of obstacles in learning the skill. Primary among them is an Inner Critic should not to initiate, which presents as related to polar type functioning. Tough partners frequently resist initiating reporting their feelings, because the Inner Critic characterizes feeling talk as "weak." Tender partners may feel reluctant to initiate because of an Inner Critic should against being "pushy" in conversations. When a Self-Sufficient partner considers initiating, the person's Inner Critic pejoritizes such assertiveness as too vulnerable. The Dependent partner does not want to offend the other and potentially lose love and connection. In each case, the person can identify the Inner Critic message and make a congruent releasing statement. For example, the Tough might say, "I have the right to look weak." The Tender can assert, "I have the right to get my agenda accepted and even to compete with others." The Self-Sufficient can challenge, "I have to right to make a mistake and be imperfect." The Dependent person can state, "I have the right to attempt to structure the conversation, even if other people don't like it. If they happen to not like it, we can negotiate."

Creating a Contract for Depth

Substantive conversations are basic to happiness and well-being (Mehl, Vazire, Holleran, & Clark, 2010). Mehl's research found that when people engage less in small talk, defined as uninvolved trivial conversations, and more in substantive conversations, involving depth connection and addressing deeper meanings and motivations, they are happier and have a greater sense of well-being. High-voltage communication comprises such substantive conversation. HVRs are essentially contractual relationships, in which both partners agree to communicate in depth utilizing skills for addressing conflict. The therapist listens for an indication from the couple that one or both partners would like more closeness, which is the opening for the therapist to double, "Is it like, I would like more depth, more closeness in our relationship?" If the partner responds affirmatively, the therapist asks for a verbal contract, "Would you each like to learn skills for creating greater closeness?" An agreement from both partners provides the foundation for beginning to teach high-voltage communication skills in context to the couple's issues. The contract also provides leverage as a value chosen by the couple when defenses triggered by increasing closeness appear.

Connecting and Focusing

A connected and focused conversation is one in which the responder's responses are directly connected to what the speaker has said. When responses are tangential, defensive, evasive, dissociated, ambiguous, indirect, or irrelevant to the topic, a *disconnect* occurs.

Connecting is one of the most important skills in maintaining the HVR. It is basic to all high voltage communications. Without it, misunderstandings occur, problems are not addressed, and minor conflicts escalate into unresolvable problems.

An important distinction is needed here. Connecting does not refer to being close, loving, or intimate. Briefly put, connecting means engaging in a focused discussion, in which each statement or question presented by one person receives a directly connected response by the other person. In other words, each person focuses on what the other has said rather than engaging in a free association response.

Following is an example of a connected conversation:

Marla: "When would you like to leave?"

Erik: "Seven p.m."

Erik's answer is direct, clear, and crisp.

Some connecting answers, while not so precise, still remain connected to the question posed:

Roberto: "When will you be ready to leave?"

Elayna: "In an hour or two."

A variation of a connected answer Elayna might have provided includes, "Well, that depends on how many sandwiches you want me to make."

While provisional in content, the answer also directly addresses the question Roberto asked.

In contrast, following are examples of disconnected responses reported in clinical sessions:

Brian: "I went to a lecture on a psychotherapy-based way of life, and the speaker said some things that were really interesting."

Brian's Mother: "Brian, let me ask you a question. What do you think heaven is like?"

Following is another example of a disconnect:

Julia: "When will you be finished with your work?"

Tony: "I don't know."

Julia: "No idea at all."

Tony: "No."

Julia: "Well, will it be in five minutes?"

Tony: "Oh, no. Not that short a time."

Julia: "Will it be in two days?"

Tony: "Oh, no. Not that long."

Julia: "Four hours?"

Tony: "What are you trying to do? Trap me?"

As the therapist helped the couple analyze what had occurred in this interchange, the intrapsychic structure fueling it became clear. As Julia began to seek a connected response from Tony, he began to evidence a self-sufficient polar type defense, in which giving a direct answer is avoided. The evasion of a direct response is employed in order to avoid feeling trapped by committing to a time frame. The therapist was able to help Tony see the Inner Critic should driving his defense: "You should not tell Julia a time frame, because if you do, you have to stick to it." Tony challenged this Inner Critic should by stating, "Just Because I tell Julia a time frame, does not mean I am trapped into doing it. I have the right to say I will be ready by a certain time and then have to renegotiate it."

Julia further lamented, "Sometimes Tony doesn't say anything to me; just sits there in silence. What do I do then?" The therapist recognized that Tony, lacking Inner Critic challenging skills, had employed what Gottman (1999) terms stonewalling. Stonewalling is a common strategy Self-Sufficient polar types often use in order to defend against the anxiety engendered by responding in a connected way. The Anthetic Relationship Therapy response the therapist taught Julia was to say, "Any response to what I just said?"

What causes disconnectedness? In clinical experience, a number of possibilities have surfaced: self-centeredness; devaluing what the other has to say; avoidance of feeling inferior when confronting issues; avoidance of Inner Critic attacks; vengeful silence for past hurts; and a choice against high-voltage communication.

If a partner frequently disconnects, the therapist may explore the cause and process the reactive structure driving it that is preventing the person from being free to connect.

Interested Questioning

Interested Questioning is essential for a successful HVR, requiring a genuine interest in the other person. Partners may employ two types of Interested Questions in their conversations. The first type, *Responsive Interested Questions,* occurs when a partner directly addresses a statement made by the speaker. For example, Gary says, "I think I blew the job interview today." Caroline responds, "Oh, what leads you to say that?" Her question indicates interest in Gary and is an overture to deeper connection.

The second type, Originary Interested Questions, is originated by the speaker. An example occurs as Gene asks, "What article were you reading in the newspaper?" Also in this category are questions evoking opinions; for example, "What do you think of X?" Originary Interested Questions may lead the conversation into even great depth when comprising quite personal questions. Examples include:

"Are you happy?"
"What do you love about me?"
"Are you feeling troubled about something?"
"Do you like or dislike the kind of questions I've been asking you?

Because Interested Questions are invitations to increase the voltage of a conversation, they may be perceived as intrusive by low-voltage partners. The response of the partner to Interested Questions is an indication of how much voltage partners desire. If both partners want high-voltage, any difficulty coping with it can be reduced by addressing fears or anxieties that arise. If the partner has not contracted for high-voltage, the partners may proceed to communicate in more surface ways that reduce the depth and intensity of the relationship.

The case of Dixie and her new husband Nathan illustrates how partners come to terms with the voltage values choice. Married three months, they consulted the Anthetic therapist for a number of problems. Dixie, a widow, had been previously married for 25 years to Bennett and had an LVR with him. Bennett was a wealthy surgeon, and he and Dixie had lived more or less parallel lives, with little involvement. Dixie stated that she did not mind too much because Bennett's income provided ample money to spend, and she had a wide circle of friends and relatives. Approximately one year after Bennett's death, she met Nathan and was impressed by how different he was from Bennett. Whereas Bennett had functioned as a Self-Sufficient type, Nathan wanted intense closeness. Dixie was delighted with his vitality but did not quite know how to handle the new situation.

At the first session, one of her complaints was that Nathan was trying to control her. "He keeps interrogating me," she said. "He asks, 'What do you think of this; what do you think of that? Where did you buy that? Do you like it? What do you like about it?' It feels like I'm getting the third degree."

Guided by the concept of voltage choice, instead of helping Dixie make a request that Nathan ask fewer questions, the therapist saw this moment as an opportunity to place before the couple a basic decision—what level of voltage they desired: high-voltage or low-voltage.

After the therapist described the two options, they both declared that they wanted high voltage. Nathan said he had married (and divorced) a woman who functioned in a low voltage way and now wanted someone who appreciated closeness and intensity. Dixie hesitated but finally chose high voltage also. However, she had become so accustomed to a low-voltage marriage where partners asked no questions of each other that the high-voltage way of relating was new and uncomfortable.

As she explored her feelings, she discovered that she had disliked questions because, as she stated, it gave other people power over her when she answered. It reminded her of how her mother used to ask her questions when she came home from a date. That was the link to the past. She was staving off what she mistakenly thought was a power giveaway by trying to legislate against the asking of questions by her new husband.

She began to realize that from the Anthetic voltage perspective, Nathan simply wanted more closeness. As soon as she was able to reframe what he was doing, she began to be open to Nathan's interested questions, and the couple enjoyed the greater involvement that occurred with the HVR.

As Dixie and Nathan illustrate, even when couples say they want high voltage, they will need new skills to handle that voltage and to cope with the intensity that couples have described as "the high gale effect"; in which partners feel the intensity of close communication as threatening to overwhelm them and to cause them to lose their balance. The balance is actually the challenge to maintain one's identity and selfhood in the face of the intensity one feels.

The chief psychological obstacle to practicing the Interested Question skill is a partner's belief that asking such questions is nosy and rude. That, the therapist points out is an Inner Critic message, trying to keep the person safe by commanding the he or she be polite and superficial and not to take any risks in getting deeper. Of course, moving deeper does indeed involve risks.

However, once the couple learns HVR skills, they benefit by the depth, intensity and increased love and affection.

Checking for Feelings

This skill is a special form of Interested Questioning. It involves one partner asking the other what he or she is feeling and consists of the words, "What are you feeling?" It is best used only when one partner is genuinely interested in discovering the other's feelings. When genuine, this skill becomes an important foundation for creating closeness. In fact, research finds that revelation of emotions, particularly vulnerable emotions such as guilt, hurt, or sadness that expresses the partner's deepest self, is an essential feature of intimate interactions (Johnson & Greenberg, 1994; Prager & Roberts, 2004; Roberts & Greenberg, 2002).

When should the couple employ this skill?

1. To discover the impact of their statements, questions, or behavior
2. To complete an interaction, tying up any loose ends
3. To discover each other's state of mind particularly if one thinks the other partner is feeling distant, depressed, hurt, or angry
4. At any time that one partner has engaged in high-voltage communication and suspects that the other partner has had some feelingful reaction to discover whether this has occurred

Frequently partners when introduced to this skill assert, "We ask each other about feelings all the time. Just this morning, I asked him, 'What's wrong?'" Their assertion points to an important lack of understanding as well as a necessary refinement in order for the couple to be skillful in checking for feelings. The therapist points out these refinements and cautions the couple to avoid saying the following:

"What's the matter?" (This implies defectiveness.) Other versions that also imply defectiveness include, "What's wrong?" "What's bothering you?" and "What's eating you?"

"What's happening?" (This form is ineffective in eliciting feelings due to its broadness and non-specificity.) In addition, the statement "A penny for your thoughts" is too indirect. Instead, the skill of Checking for Feelings is best used in one of the following versions:

- "What are you feeling?" (This is the recommended form.)
- "What are you feeling right now?" (This is also recommended as it is more focused.)
- "What did you feel when I said that?" (This is a good variant.)
- "Did you have any feelings while I was talking?" (This is another good variant.)
- A few good shorthand forms of the skill include: "Any feelings?" "Are you OK?" "Where are you psychologically?"

An important refinement to the skill is that partners are recommended to ask, "*What* are you feeling?" not "*How* are you feeling?" as the latter is a colloquial form that tends to elicit a ritualistic response of "Fine."

Much of everyday conversation consists of "story." People tell stories about their activities, plans, decisions, accomplishments, projects, hopes, and various events that have happened to them. Engaging in "story" can be called Level 1. No feelings are reported. Conversations are similar to news stories where happenings are reported. This level provides partners with surface connection and is a valuable first step in revealing what each has experienced.

However, in order to create the deeper connection of high-voltage communication, partners can shift the level of conversation by asking after an event is reported, "What did you feel when that happened?" Doing so facilitates Level 2 connection, consisting of *feelings* about happenings.

For partners who wish to deepen the level of connection even further (Level 3), one can ask the other, "What were you feeling about me while I was talking to you?" One more deepening can occur (Level 4) when partners learn to ask, "Have you had any feelings toward me that you haven't mentioned yet?"

To summarize, Level 1 comprises reporting of events; Level 2 elicits feelings about those events; Level 3 evokes feelings that partners have toward each other in the moment; and Level 4 elicits feelings that may be hidden and withheld. As partners learn to move deeper using the elicitation skills, voltage intensifies. In order to tolerate and then enjoy the depth they are achieving, partners must be taught to pair these interchanges with skills for challenging any Inner Critic messages that are triggered by the intensity of the communication.

Accessing and Reporting Feelings

In order to respond to the skills of Checking for Feelings, each partner must possess skill in accessing and reporting feelings. Accessing feelings refers to being able to get in touch with or identify feelings. For partners who have difficulty identifying their feelings, the therapist can guide them by asking, "Did you feel good or bad?" Partners are almost always able to provide this basic identification of feelings. Once this gross assessment is provided, the therapist can offer a number of options within the category of good or bad in order to help partners specify feelings; for example, "Did you feel angry, sad, hurt?"

Following Accessing feelings by identifying them, partners can deepen connection by Reporting feelings to each other. The therapist teaches the couple that Reporting feelings requires knowledge of an important distinction. Reporting means talking about the feeling. The feeling then becomes an element in the partner's mind. In contrast, acting out the feeling means dramatizing the feeling in actions. When acting out a feeling, the person mentally fuses with it so that it becomes a state of mind that is then expressed instrumentally, in order to have an impact on the partner. An example of acting out is "You're a stupid idiot!" An example of Reporting is "I feel angry at you."

Reporting feelings is a skill for producing involvement, facilitating empathy, identifying dysfunctional areas on which to work, and noting when emotionality is seeping into the rational part of the psyche. Acting out feelings is destructive to closeness.

The value of the skill of accessing and reporting feelings is manifold for the following reasons:

1. Feelings are the avenue to personal growth. As partners identify a feeling, then follow with an archeological dig into layers beneath; they are able to analyze and evaluate the feeling.
2. Knowing one's feelings and then evaluating them in the light of what the Natural Self desires facilitate decision-making and effective pursuit of goals.
3. Awareness of one's feelings equips the person with the self-knowledge necessary to decrease vulnerability to pressure and verbal attacks from others.
4. The more proficient partners become in Accessing and Reporting feelings, the more opportunities occur for deeper and more satisfying relationships.
5. As partners are able to access feelings, they gain the benefit of identifying twinges of pain when someone has targeted them with judgmentalism or anger.
6. Reporting a feeling is an important step in taking distance from it, so it no longer drives behavior, thus breaking the reactive mechanism of automatically acting out a feeling; for example, "If I feel angry at someone, I've got to get revenge" or "If I feel guilty about something, I've got to explain and defend myself."
7. Partners are able to engage in argument analysis. For example, a partner can report, "Oh, just before I got angry at you, I felt hurt."

8. Partners become skillful in answering each other's question, "What are you feeling?"

   In summary, the skill of accessing and reporting feelings is essential in producing an HVR.

Following are steps the therapist teaches regarding the skill of Accessing and Reporting Feelings:

1. First, slow things down. Relax. Be silent for a moment or two. Take enough time to check inside. Deliberately interrupt and bracket any automatic, machinelike processes or thoughts that are going on inside.
2. Rather than look for a bodily felt sense ("My stomach feels tight"), look for an emotion ("I feel scared").
3. Introspect. Look inside.
4. Identify a feeling, no matter how faint, seemingly inappropriate, improper, or excessive it seems.
5. Disregard the Inner Critic's messages that the feelings are petty, not valid, and inappropriate.
6. Report the feeling, beginning with the words "I feel" and ending with the name of a feeling ("angry," "loving," "suspicious," or "depressed").
7. Avoid reporting transitive feelings that contain implied accusations of one's partner. Transitive feeling reports usually begin with the words "I feel like." Examples include, "I feel like I'm being judged" or "I feel like I'm being rejected." Instead report, "I feel guilty" or "I feel hurt." If partners think the other is being judgmental or rejecting, they can offer that information as feedback. Feedback can include questions such as "Are you feeling judgmental?" or "Are you feeling distant?"

As the therapist teaches these steps, a number of psychological obstacles may surface in the couple. Most contain dysfunctional learning from parents or the culture. Examples include "Big boys don't cry"; "You have no reason to feel depressed"; "Settle down. Don't get so excited"; "Don't be such a scaredy-cat"; "I know you're feeling bad that he's died, but he wouldn't want you to cry about it"; and "Don't wear your heart on your sleeve."

In order to assist partners in becoming free from such legislative injunctions against feelings, the therapist can guide them in challenging the Inner Critic which has internalized the messages. Such Inner Critic challenging is essential throughout the learning process, because partners will have Inner Critic material that can block their learning or practicing of this skill. Many of these will be consistent with each partner's polar type. Tough partners will have shoulds not to express or even have tender feelings. Tender partners will labor under shoulds not to trigger pain in others by expressing anger or hurt. Self-sufficient partners may have shoulds not to identify or express feelings of neediness. Dependent partners will have shoulds not to be impolite or to hurt others by being honest or blunt about their feelings.

Being Forthcoming: Self-Disclosure

Much of high-voltage communication has self-disclosure at its heart. Self-disclosure refers to talking about oneself; not only reporting feelings but also giving opinions, expressing thoughts, declaring who one is, revealing one's likes and dislikes, revelation of one's life happenings, and announcing one's hopes and plans. Like Interested Questions, self-disclosure can be originary or responsive.

Psychological obstacles to practicing this skill have their origin in the Inner Critic. They include:

1. Beliefs no one would be interested
2. Fear of criticism, humiliation, or rejection
3. Aversion to becoming involved with others
4. Beliefs that talking about oneself is egotistical, self-centered, or arrogant
5. Mistrust of others response to one's self-revelation, including using the information against one.

Quotidian Honesty

Standard relationships often are conducted on a low-voltage level. They are guided by the rule of avoiding upsetting others through honesty, self-revelation, or requesting. In contrast, HVRs are based upon quotidian honesty involving speaking honestly about one's feelings and preferences, as well as one's dislikes.

Partners may at first resist this skill due to similar psychological obstacles that surface when learning to be forthcoming. Partners fear offending or hurting others, appearing arrogant or neurotic, creating an argument, and becoming the target of retaliation.

In each case, the therapist poses to partners the basic values choice. Do they choose an HVR or an LVR? While there might be repercussions, these can be processed. In such moments, partners have the opportunity to integrate personal growth methods with relationship skills. One important advantage of the use of the skill of quotidian honesty is an increase in trust or restoration of trust in partners.

Vulnerability Talk

Feelings appear in layers; the top layers serve a defensive function. Many couples speak and act from these layers, including "story," making acquittal statements, and acting on impulses to withdraw. The purpose of the defensive layers is to protect the person against Inner Critic pain. Living from this layer has a detrimental effect of building walls and enforcing low-voltage relating.

Underneath these defensive-distancing layers is usually a negativity layer comprising feelings such as anger and judgmentalism. The negativity layer serves a protective function against emotional pain but does so by defending against the underlying layer of vulnerability.

Vulnerability talk includes talking about feelings of fear, hurt, being gypped, shame, guilt, neediness, and other items that the Inner Critic would condemn. Speaking from the vulnerability layer seems risky to partners, because it opens them to the possibility of criticism and other forms of negativity. In addition, engaging in such talk opens each partner to becoming conscious of feelings about which they may have previously been unconscious. Nevertheless, vulnerability talk forms the solid foundation for HVRs.

As couples gain the interpersonal skills to begin to create connection, closeness increases. With each foray into greater closeness, the probability of triggering emotional pain increases, as does the need for skills for handling defensive negativity.

Chapter 9

Interpersonal Skills for Handling Negativity in Relationships

The intensity of intimate relationships creates myriad opportunities for partners' negative thoughts, emotions, and behaviors to arise. In what feels like the strong gale of such negativity, partners employ a variety of strategies in order to cope. Kouneski and Olson's (2004) ENRICH typology (based on a randomized sample of 10,000 couples) classifies couples as either stable or unstable. Stable couples (those exhibiting greater closeness) range in intimacy from vitalized (the most emotionally connected and the most skilled in resolving conflict; 21%) to harmonious (somewhat skilled in conflict resolution; 11%) to traditional (those embedded in external social support but with less closeness between partners; 14%). Unstable couples; those with less intimacy and greater distress were grouped in two types, that is, conflicted (exhibiting more controlling and avoidant behaviors; 25%) and devitalized (discouraged and with less motivation and skill in conflict resolution; 29%) (Kouneski, 2002). Unstable couples (54% of the sample) displayed the distress, criticism, and contempt observed by Gottman (1993) in his research on distressed couples and exhibited the highest risk for divorce.

In light of such research findings, a clear need exists for innovative interventions to help couples who enter intimate relationships with hope of happiness, achieve closeness and satisfaction. This chapter describes the high-voltage communication and Relationship skills (the interpersonal skills) that over forty years of clinical application, have helped couples, both those with severe distress as well as those who function well but want to sustain closeness, to reinvent their relationships as a safe haven. These skills equip couples to achieve emotional closeness not merely once in a while, but rather in everyday conversations. They provide skills for partners to do troubleshooting when conflict occurs. This chapter offers word-for-word scripts therapists can teach couples to achieve optimal relationships for a lifetime.

Application of the Lament and the Anthetic Sacrament for Negativity Reduction

Partners seeking therapy typically enter in a great deal of emotional pain. As described in Chapter 8, the Anthetic Relationship Therapy approach views directly addressing emotional pain as the first item in the therapeutic protocol. Emotional pain will demand attention and continue to evidence itself until attended to. The therapist's initial task is to listen for each partner's expression of pain. The lament is defined as a cry of pain and can be identified by a variety of partner behaviors. For example, a person may express a lament through tears, complaints, anger, blame, or even silent withdrawal. It is imperative that the therapist attend as quickly as possible to each partner's lament with empathy. By the time couples seek therapy, their laments have often gone unheard by each other, and even when heard, have, due to lack of skill, become magnified in their expression in an attempt to have them attended to.

Anthetic Relationship Therapy offers the skill of the anthetic sacrament by which the therapist guides partners to offer to each other. To clarify, the term "sacrament" here is not meant to imply a religious sacrament, but rather a psychological and spiritual one. As partners offer each other the deep empathy contained in this communication, a sacred space opens, and partners report a flow of love for each other that has a transcendent quality; one that prior to offering it was unforeseeable, given the pain the partners were experiencing. The following form for the Anthetic Sacrament is a word-for-word script the therapist guides partners to say to each other in response to a lament:

- "I'm so sorry that you are having this pain." The therapist clarifies that the words, "I'm so sorry," are not an apology but rather a statement of deep empathy similar to words said at a funeral, when a person tells the bereaved, "I'm so sorry for your loss." No responsibility or guilt is implied.
- "You didn't deserve that. What you deserved was ______________." In clinical reports from couples, this statement holds great solace to the person experiencing pain. One explanation may be that interpersonal pain often contains an element of failure of expectation of a response of caring or love, whether the pain had its source in the partner, a relative, a co-worker, or a stranger.

In review of clinical application of the skill of identifying laments and offering the anthetic sacrament with hundreds of couples, two benefits appear regarding research in the literature on negativity in couples. Because partners learn a concept for quickly recognizing emotional pain in each other, the negativity threshold is lowered (see Gottman, 1999, p. 73–74), providing protection against chronic escalating negative responding to one another. Second, the therapist, rather than being the *soother* to both partners, teaches the partners to soothe one another by offering deep empathy through the anthetic sacrament. This is consistent with the finding by Gottman (1999) that upon termination of therapy, therapeutic gains erode, because the therapist had fulfilled the role of soother and de-escalator. Through the skill of the anthetic sacrament, which is a simple brief script, partners can soothe each other while in diffuse physiological arousal. In addition, the empathy engendered in the skill creates a climate of a safe haven from which partners can address the specific content of their needs and wants.

Anthetic Requesting

Following the expression of empathy contained in the Anthetic Sacrament, the therapist will most often introduce the second interpersonal skill that is foundational to optimal relating, that is, anthetic requesting. The indication for teaching this skill occurs when partners voice a complaint, anger, or judgmentalism. Upon hearing any of these indicators, the therapist states, "I'd like to teach you a skill for more effectively getting what you want from each other. It is the anthetic requesting skill." The therapist then offers a handout with the eight-step skill and guides the partners in making the request that was contained in the complaint or other negative statement and states, "I'd like you to use these steps word for word until you have mastered them. After that, you can experiment with changes:"

1. "I have a request that you…"
2. "Is it clear what I'm asking?"
3. "Is it likely I'll get what I want?"
4. If the answer is a clear "Yes," ask, "Will this be easy or hard to do?"
5. If the answer is "Easy," the process is complete, and you might say "Thank you."
6. If the answer is "Hard," you'll need to do some troubleshooting. For example, "Can you say what will be hard about it?"
7. You may want to ask, "Is there any way I can help you make it easier?"
8. You may need to negotiate.

In clinical experience with thousands of couples, the Anthetic Requesting Process has brought about a dramatic reduction in defensiveness and negativity. The benefit appears to center upon the neutrality of the language in Step One, converting emotion-laden words to neutral language; the question asking for clarity in Step Two, in which previously tacit material becomes explicit; the focused communication in Step Three, normally neglected by most couples who do not ask for a response to requests; the elicitation of barriers in Steps Four, Five and Six, so that emotional or practical blocks can be surfaced; and the collaborative nature of the offer of help in Step Seven.

Making Power Differential Corrections

A power differential occurs when one person has more personal power than another. Power differentials may occur because one person actually does have power over another, and the lower-power person cannot easily escape from that power, such as in the cases of parents and children, bosses and employees, and teachers and students. More easily correctable situations include the following:

- One partner is Tough and assertive; the other is Tender and self-effacing (see Chapter 3)
- One partner has more power through achieving more inner freedom by doing extensive work on becoming free of his or her Inner Critic
- One partner may have more money than the other
- One partner may attempt to control another through emotional means; for example, anger, crying, or judgmentalism
- One partner may attempt to control another through a facial expression denoting disapproval, suspiciousness, or scorn
- One person has power conferred by the culture, while the other person is disempowered by commands that come from the culture and that are incorporated into the less powerful person's Inner Critic

Even if the relationship is a high-voltage one, chosen by both partners, there still may be a power differential. This is often difficult for the higher power partner to realize. Self-centeredness may lead that person to think that everyone is able to be as assertive as he or she is. Therefore, this disempowerment, if it exists, must be admitted by both partners and discussed openly, with solutions negotiated. The following are questions the higher power partner can ask in order to correct the power differential:

- "Are you doing exactly what you want to be doing?"
- "Are you afraid of having an opinion or preference that is different from mine?"
- "Did you agree to that just to please me?"
- "Are you having a should?"
- "I hope my crying/anger/judgmentalism doesn't put any pressure on you to do something. Are you feeling pressure? Can you resist it? I don't want you

to be pushed around by my feelings. Can you make a releasing statement so you can get free? An example is, 'Just because you're crying doesn't mean I have to do a thing.'"
- "I feel a pull to try to control you, but my bottom line is I want you to be free. I don't want you to be controlled by my feelings."

In listening to the answers to these questions, the therapist, as well as the partner with greater power should be aware that certain phrases are indicative of a self-disempowered attitude. Examples include, "I guess so"; "Whatever you want"; and "It doesn't matter to me."

In order to correct the power differential and support the less powerful partner in exercising power, the greater power person will need to engage consistently in checking one or more times to ensure the partner is operating from a free choice.

Switching Out of Coercive Controllingness

Usually observed in Tough partners, coercive controllingness consists of a desperate and self-centered attempt to dominate the relationship or otherwise control the behavior of other people. This strategy indicates a lack of interest in the partner's inner freedom along with an over-concern with need fulfillment at any cost. It can take the form of angry forcefulness or micromanagement through careful monitoring of the partner. When its roots are explored in therapy, the subconscious theme in coercive control is an inability to tolerate anxiety when not in control. It most often has its roots in childhood learning. In therapy, the person who relies on coercive control can gain skills for reducing anxiety and tolerating negative affect (Chapter 7), along with Inner Critic challenging (Chapter 3) and Inner Figure orchestration (Chapter 4). The process can be accelerated through feedback the controller elicits through the request, "Please tell me every time you see me doing something that's controlling."

Processing One's Own Negativity

Negativity is the most common obstacle to achieving an HVR. It consists of several related and overlapping processes, including demonizing, discounting, blaming, ignoring, and displaying anger and harsh criticism. In order to process negativity, the person first asks for feedback from his or her partner: "Tell me every time you see or hear me being negative." (In order to tolerate such feedback, the person will need to employ Inner Critic challenging skills.) Upon hearing the feedback, the person then substitutes the anthetic requesting process for the negativity.

Anthetic Listening

Anthetic listening is distinguished from ordinary social conversation. In social conversation, first one person talks about himself or herself, then the other responds with talk about himself. In addition, anthetic listening is distinguished from problem-plus-advice talk. Here one person presents a problem, while the other person offers advice or a possible solution.

In contrast, anthetic listening is more structured. One person does almost all the talking, while the second person does most of the listening and limits his or her responses to those that will be helpful in creating space in which the first person can think and talk. A technique drawn from psychotherapy, anthetic listening takes the simple form of the listener asking, "Can you tell me more about that?"

The skill does not include mirroring; the paraphrasing often recommended by communication skills trainers, in which the listener offers a second person reflection summarizing what the speaker has said.

The therapist teaches partners to respond with the anthetic listening question no matter what the other has said; even if the partner has said something highly charged (e.g., "I want to move to Alaska"; "I think we should have a baby"; or "Let's go into business for ourselves."

In creating an optimal relationship, anthetic listening is essential. It equips partners to facilitate emotional closeness by skillfully handling such feedback as, "You seem distant; "I don't like the way our relationship is going"; "I've been thinking of leaving you"; or "I'm not sure I'm still in love with you." In each case, the response, "Can you tell me more about that" opens conversation to reveal more fully what a partner is thinking or feeling, at which point partners can apply further skills.

The therapist teaches the couple to ask for or clarify a contract. Ideally, when one partner would like to talk about a problem, he or she asks, "Can you do some anthetic listening?" If the other partner responds with "Yes," a contract exists. However, at times, partners may not be explicit and instead begin with a statement such as, "I'm feeling some fear about the speech I'm supposed to give." When this occurs, the partner needs to offer the two kinds of contract by asking "Do you want me to just listen, or would you like some advice?" In other words, the therapist helps partners understand that the mention of a problem does not imply an automatic assumption that the person wants help solving the problem. He or she may simply want to explore it out loud while the partner listens and/or asks questions. Similarly, partners must not automatically assume that the other wants anthetic listening. He or she may want some advice. Checking with each other using the checking out assumptions skill will reveal their wishes.

Following is a typical anthetic listening conversation between partners:

Finn: "Mom has been so forgetful lately. I'm afraid she might be developing Alzheimer's."

Desi: "Can you tell me more about that?"

Finn explores further, and as she pauses, Desi asks: "Anything else?"

When Finn says, "No, nothing else," Desi says, "Thank you for telling me."

Finally, Desi does Research about his listening. "Was what I did helpful?" If Finn says, Yes, Desi can probe further and ask, "How was it helpful?" He might also ask, "Did I do anything that was not helpful?"

At this point, the anthetic listening session is complete and if they choose, the couple can return to social conversation mode. Alternatively, they may switch to a problem-solving or advice-giving mode. The session might also have stirred up some feelings in the listening partner who may request anthetic listening.

Certain blocks to anthetic listening can emerge in couples, including difficulty focusing on another person due to impulsiveness, self-centeredness, or a pattern of coercive control. In such instances, the therapist can assist that partner with skills mentioned previously.

Partners find that practicing anthetic listening reaps surprising benefits. For example, they may find out new elements in their partner's thinking, feeling, or personality they had not previously known. For partners who overvalue advice-giving, hearing feedback on how valuable just listening was may be enlightening and lead to a pattern of greater flexibility in speaking and listening. In addition, the speaker may learn how useful this method is for processing thoughts and feelings without being concerned about fending off criticism, interruptions, or advice-giving.

Interruption Skills

While for many people, any interruption seems disrespectful and dysfunctional, clinical observation of thousands of couples, has revealed that some interruptions are necessary for constructive discussion. These include emergency interruptions ("What's that burning smell?"); physical process interruptions ("Let me interrupt you. I have to leave in about five minutes. Can we agree to continue our discussion later?"); emotional process interruptions ("Let me interrupt you. You seem to be getting very angry. I'd like you to process your anger before we continue"); non-understanding interruptions ("I'm not understanding what you're saying"); and anti-repetitiousness interruptions ("Let me interrupt you. I think you told me this yesterday. Unless you have some new additions"). In the last situation, the partner who is being repetitious may respond, "I know I said this yesterday, but I just want to go over it to get clear in my mind" or "I realize I said these things yesterday, but I just want to savor them."

While the above interruptions are generally constructive, some may be disruptive. One category consists of self-centeredness-based interruptions, in which the person attempts to change the topic in midstream to one that is more satisfying to the interrupter. Another category includes impatience-based interruptions. These often occur in response to a question about which the interrupter feels too impatient to hear fully. A third category consists of corrective interruptions designed to "correct the record." One partner reported in therapy that he felt driven to correct anything his partner said that contradicted the facts he felt were true, and so he continually interrupted her.

In order to help couples make interruptions constructively, the therapist can guide them in signaling their intent, primarily by saying, "Let me interrupt you." The purpose of the signal is to announce a change of topic. The listener then has the option of accepting or rejecting the interruption. However, one option available to the speaker is, "Let me lay this whole thing out before you respond."

Switching Out of Defensiveness and Touchiness

When given feedback of any kind, partners may be driven to defend, explain, justify, and essentially get acquitted. Partners report that the impulse seems like an absolute necessity; something they are compelled to do. The explanation lies in the person's pride in living up to a compensatory self-image that defends against Inner Critic condemnation. By defending, partners miss the opportunity for handling feedback in a task-oriented way that has the potential to lead to freedom and growth. A pattern of defensiveness is consistent with negative sentiment override found by Gottman (1999) to lead partners to misperceive communications as hostile or attacking. Because negative sentiment override is associated with failure in conflict resolution, couples aspiring to optimal HVRs must be given skills for becoming free from it.

In Anthetic Relationship Therapy, the therapist can offer four possible self-statements in order to help partners get free and accordingly be equipped to consider any feedback carefully:

1. "I don't have to defend myself."
2. "I choose not to defend myself."
3. "I have a pull to defend myself, but I'm not going to act on it."
4. "I have a pull to defend myself, but I'm not going to go there."

Anthetic Conflict Resolution

Conflicts occur because people have differing values, desires, and attitudes. Because partners in HVR aspire to a significantly greater degree of closeness than LVRs, these differences may surface even more frequently. In the area of couple conflict, Anthetic Relationship Therapy agrees with Gottman (1999) that what is needed is *dialogue* about the conflict. However, this approach offers hope for what Gottman labeled perpetual and gridlocked problems. Clinical work with couples over the last forty years indicates that the following protocol can equip partners with the skills needed to resolve conflict, even those that have been cyclical and repetitive for the couple. The therapist can lead partners through this process during couple sessions, and then provide them with these steps to use at home.

1. Go over the Anthetic Dialogue of ideas (Chapter 12)
2. Make any value shifts that are necessary, especially a shift to the value of rationality (Chapter 6), along with the value of pleasure
3. If necessary, recover from any self-centeredness (Chapter 7)
4. Address and process all negativity, with partners taking turns giving each other feedback about negativity, using the methods in this chapter for eliminating negativity
5. Make any power differential corrections that may be needed (this chapter)
6. Switch out of controllingness (this chapter)
7. Identify and disentangle any responsibility tangles (this chapter)
8. Most important, use the conflict as an occasion to work on becoming individuated, that is, partners' disengaging from enmeshment with each other (Chapter 7)
9. Partners assess their readiness to resolve the conflict, based on whether they have completed the above steps

Having completed all nine steps, each partner should now be in the correct state of mind to engage in task-oriented discussion, that is, discussion focused rationally on the tasks to be done rather than being contaminated by emotional seepage.

The therapist can then guide partners through the next steps having to do with negotiation and decision making, after which partners may use the steps independently of the therapist on future conflict:

- First, partners make a clear statement of the issue involved. For example, "Where should we go on vacation this year?"
- Second, partners list the criteria each holds for a possible choice. For example, "It must be near water, inexpensive, and have good restaurants

nearby." Each partner should then rate each criterion on a scale of 0 (not important) to 10 (very important).

- Third, partners make a list of all possible items that might satisfy the criteria. Evaluate each item with regard to the criteria listed above.
- Fourth, each partner may choose one item after another, then rate it as to desirability on a scale of zero to ten. Following this, each person can rate the partner's choice as to undesirability, on a scale of negative ten to zero. Partners can then compare scale values. In general, it is a good idea to reject any proposed solution if either partner has a strong negative scale value for it.
- Fifth, partners explore compromises. For example, partners could spend part of their vacation at one place and part at another place.
- Sixth, partners explore the possibility of making a decision only as an experiment. For example, partners make the choice provisionally, with the option of discontinuing it immediately if it leads to a high negative scale value for either partner.
- Seventh, partners ask how well the decision making went. Could anything be improved?

As partners proceed with the therapist's help through each of previous steps, any emotional reactivity can be reported and the appropriate skill applied. The protocol thus is to attend to reactivity first; then return to rational decision-making.

Initiating Reconciliations

Relational conflict occurs even in the best of HVRs. Partners may feel hurt, abandoned, or betrayed, whereupon they withdraw, physically and/or emotionally. What is needed at that time is the skill of *initiating a reconciliation.* To do so one partner must actively pursue the other. Such pursuit requires a value shift to valuing closeness, love, and a safe haven over acting out pain through revenge or distancing.

Steps in practicing this skill follow:

1. The first step consists of a partner deciding whether the relationship is important to him or her.
2. The second step consists of a request: "Can we talk about such-and-such?" If the partner says "No," that is an example of extreme distancing and a choice for low voltage. If this occurs during a therapy session, the therapist can do focused individual work on the element that has led to the surfacing of any rigid defense. If the partner does not want to engage in this work, the therapist can simply ask if the partner is satisfied with the level

of closeness and draw any ramifications regarding the couple's intimacy entailed in this choice.

3. If the partner says Yes to the request for talking, the third step is the reconciliation itself. The therapist may begin by checking for feelings. Each then labels any reactivity about which he or she is aware, following which each processes the reactivity using the appropriate skill. Finally each can be helped to declare a resolution to do things differently next time. The therapist can ask (and teach the couple to ask each other), "How would you have liked that to have gone?"

One obstacle to Initiating a Reconciliation is pride. The statement, "I'm not going to be the one who goes first," indicates that a partner has fused with his or her reactive pride system. Having identified this process, the therapist can point out the Inner Critic's influence and assist the person in making a releasing statement: "I have the right to go first, even though my Inner Critic is telling me that it would be humiliating and a sign of weakness."

Retrieval and Repair Skills

Gottman's research (1999) on the importance of repair attempts led him to recommend that couple therapy only be considered successful when couples are capable of repair independently of the therapist. Hence, Anthetic Relationship Therapy offers the couple skills to use to accomplish their own repair of hurt and conflict.

Partners often experience the mistakes they make as devastating. The therapist can help by pointing out that any feelings of devastation are merely the Inner Critic functioning to deliver emotional punishments in the form of feelings of defectiveness, guilt, shame, inferiority, or magnified fear. Following this labeling, the therapist can assist the person with a challenge to the Inner Critic in the form of a releasing statement; for example, "I have the right to make mistakes, even a thousand mistakes. I have the right to be an imperfect partner."

In addition to the intrapersonal Inner Critic work, the partner may also use any of the following interpersonal statements for the purpose of retrieval of the situation:

- "Cancel what I just said."
- "You know the thing I said this morning? I take it back. Here's my real bottom-line position."
- "About what I said: That was just my stuff; my emotional baggage."
- "Let's each process our stuff."

Couples frequently ask, "Is it a good idea to apologize?" The therapist can respond that they may apologize if they wish, but that apologies are not as effective as retrievals. Couples can decide if they see apologies as a form of soothing or if they choose to include them in the retrieval process. It is essential, however, that couples not rely solely on apologies for several reasons. First, apologies tend to become mechanical and meaningless. Second, apologies may tend to be relied upon as a panacea while continuing the offensive behavior. A third problem with an apology is that it may form the foundation for a new argument; for example, "You said you were sorry, but you didn't really mean it." Finally, an apology implies that the apologizer is bad, an implication contaminated by Inner Critic messages. If partners ask the therapist, "What do you do if you don't apologize?" The therapist should answer, "You say, 'That was just my stuff' (indicating emotional material on which to work). "And then you work on the material using one or more of the intrapersonal skills."

Reaching Out

Partners who follow a low-voltage style of functioning live self-encapsulated lives, often blocked by the impediments of pride and fear. In order to increase closeness and raise the voltage, partners must learn to reach out to one another. A reach-out occurs when a partner overcomes pride and fear and reaches for connection with the other person. One example of reaching out is contained in the skill of Initiating a Conversation described in Chapter 8. Another is asking an interested question. Still others are expressing positivity (Chapter 10) and Initiating a Reconciliation covered earlier in this chapter. However, anthetic relationship therapy suggests still more examples:

- Offering to shake hands or to hug
- Touching one's partner's shoulder or arm
- Asking "Can we talk about such-and-such?"
- Approaching one's partner with the question, "Mind if I join you?"
- Writing a note or letter to the other partner
- Asking one's partner for help

For some people, reaching out can feel scary. The fear is engendered as reaching out leads one to feel vulnerable to rejection. The therapist can teach someone facing this fear to make a releasing statement such as, "I have the right to reach out to this person" or "If I'm rejected, it won't be the end of the world, and they'll be missing out on connection with a good person; namely me."

Responding to Reach-Outs

For partners who desire more optimal relating, a welcoming response to reach-outs is essential. Accepting a reach-out is usually a great delight, one that will give both partners pleasure. Some options for responding include an expression of welcoming such as "Mmm. That feels good that you're reaching out to me" or "Aww. I'd love to have you join me." If the person who receives the reach-out is absorbed in a task but would like to respond, he or she can say, "I would love to join you (or talk with you). I just have to finish this task and will be ready to join you in 15 minutes."

Disentangling Responsibility Tangles

Recall from Chapter 3 the process whereby the Inner Critic demands that a person take responsibility for other's negative feelings and that a person hold others responsible for his or her own negative feelings. Taking responsibility for others' negative feelings results in a responsibility tangle. Such negative feelings include depression, fear, anger, hurt, and judgmentalism. Statements that exemplify responsibility tangles include "You made me angry" and "You put me on the defensive." In each case, this position is a form of self-disempowerment on the part of the speaker, putting him or her in the victim position, which is not conducive to an HVR. (For the same reason, the Anthetic Relationship Therapy form for elicitation of feelings is not "How did that make you feel?" Instead the therapist asks, "What did you feel when he said that" or "What did you feel when that happened?"

In order to disentangle a responsibility tangle, three skills are needed:

1. "A" makes a position statement, saying to "B," "I don't hold you responsible for my negative feelings."
2. Whenever "A" has a negative feeling, he or she uses a "when" statement instead of a "made" statement; that is, instead of saying "You made me angry because you questioned my veracity," "A" says "I felt angry when you questioned my veracity."
3. "A" uses the word "triggered" rather than "made"; that is, "You triggered my hurt feelings when you critiqued my writing."

Partners may speak honestly to one another by using reports of feelings, not "act-outs." For example, a partner may say, "I felt hurt when you said that" instead of "How *could* you have said that terrible thing to me!" Armed with this new perspective, each partner becomes responsible for his or her own feelings and can then apply skills to dismantle any reactive driving mechanism for the feelings. For example, a partner who becomes angry can work on discovering any driving factors such as Inner Critic messages or unfulfilled needs, then use the skill of Anthetic Requesting to neutrally ask for what he or she wants.

Clinical experience suggests that couples often find the land mine metaphor useful in obtaining this new perspective. In relaying this metaphor, the therapist tells the couple, "I want to offer you a metaphor for understanding responsibility tangles. It's as though we are all sown with land mines. They were put in place by old hurts from some earlier time in our lives. If our partner happens to poke the land mine, it will explode. So, any negative feeling is a clue that a land mine has been triggered and exploded. From this perspective, you can see that any given behavior may explode one person's land mine but wouldn't affect another, because he or she wouldn't have a land mine about that issue." As partners accept this new perspective, each retrieves some of the personal responsibility for his or her own feelings, along with the power to become free from idiosyncratic emotional pain.

Chapter 10

Increasing the Voltage

Depth Connecting Skills

The quote cited in the introduction of the book is worth repeating here as it illustrates an important voltage element: "Inside each person is a great reservoir of magical energies for loving in a deep way, even in a mythic way" (adapted from Elliott, K., & Elliott, J., 2014). This adaptation of the authors' memoir of love letters expresses what research indicates: Couples have the capacity for deep intimacy and emotional connection that flexibly weathers stress and transitions and leads to vitalization of their relationship (Kouneski & Olson, 2004). Given the empirical research that points to couples' capacity for optimality, the field of couple therapy needs innovative strategies for helping couples achieve increased satisfaction and intimacy (Prager, 2000). The Anthetic Relationship Therapy approach of the HVR model offers eight skills for deepening connections and thereby increasing the voltage the couple enjoys.

Beholding

In research on closeness and intimacy, researchers have found a primary path through which partners achieve closeness; that is, through partners perceiving that the central, core, and defining features of each are being both attended to and reacted to in a supportive manner (Reis, Clark, & Holmes, 2004). Psychoanalytic theories have pointed to the universal human need to be seen, acknowledged, and valued which begins in infancy but continues across the life span. Object relations approaches have theorized that central to a child's development is the ability of parents and other caregivers to accurately assess the needs of an infant. The self concepts the child develops in response to such interactions have a profound impact on later interpersonal functioning

(Baldwin, 1992). A compelling argument for the importance of caregiver responsiveness on the person is attachment theory (Bowlby, 1969/1982). As the child receives responses from others, an internal working model of self-in-relation-to-others forms. Later research on the impact of infant and childhood experiences point to the development of expectations for adult romantic relationships (Baldwin, 1992; Collins, 1996).

While partners naturally may reciprocally attend and react supportively to one another, many partners come to therapy having fallen into a pattern of merely glancing at one another. Glancing means seeing the other briefly and sketchily; taking in only the surface of the other; not seeing the other as a real person with thoughts, feelings, and needs of his or her own. The partner may be seen through an impersonal lens or as a mere source of supplies of approval or listening. Beholding, on the other hand means seeing one's partner with awe, amazement, and involvement.

Anthetic Relationship Therapy offers partners the skill of *beholding* in order to help couples consciously increase the likelihood a pattern of reciprocity will be established. Anthetic Relationship Therapy defines beholding as seeing another in depth without judgmentalism. It further includes contemplating the other; considering with respect what the beholder has observed. Beholding culminates in an attitude of hallowing, which means holding as sacred the essence that makes the person who they are. In doing this, the beholder creates an environment of safety and extreme pleasure for the one beheld to express who they are. As partners reciprocally behold one another, a depth of closeness emerges.

Anthetic Relationship Therapy offers couples a Four-Step Beholding Process:

- Step 1: Observe. In the initial step, one partner notices the other in great detail. The beholder may find it helpful to mentally scan categories such as the partner's physical characteristics, behaviors, emotional tone, intellectual functioning, spiritual life, sexual ways of being, and interpersonal interactions. At times beholding may pertain to a partner's spontaneous behavior; at other times beholding occurs following the skill of Interested Questions; or beholding may occur as the beholder views ordinary routines afresh.
- Step 2: Contemplate. The second step involves the beholder considering with respect, awe, and/or amazement what he or she sees in the partner. As the beholder pays attention to what is noticed, a new perspective of the partner will emerge. A new valuing of the partner can begin.
- Step 3: Give Partner Feedback. As the beholder communicates the contemplation of Step 2 in words, he or she can be guided by the sentence stem, "What I love about you is. . . ."

For example, the beholder observes the partner eating dinner and says, "I love how you savor your food. I love to watch you eat." Alternatively, in witnessing the partner's emotional pain, the beholder might say, "I can see how hurt you feel by what your dad said; I hate to see him treat you like that." One variation of Step 3 may occur when the beholder notices when the partner is suffering emotionally but does not know the source and asks, "Are you feeling troubled?"

- Step 4: Asking for a Response to Being Beheld. A deepening of the voltage occurs as the beholder asks, "What feelings do you have about what I've said?" Responses might include, "That feels so good to have you see me. I love your making much over me about things I do, like how I eat." Alternatively, a response might be, "Thank you for seeing my pain. I feel so comforted. No one in my family ever said a thing when Dad talked to me like that."

ANIMUS BLESSING OR ANIMA BLESSING

Among the profound findings on couples who have been labeled *masters of marriage* is a quality of everyday marital interactions that produces a climate of deep, meaningful positivity (Gottman, 1999, pp. 108–110). The HVR model offers a skill based on adding deep, soulful, and meaningful interactions between couples called the *animus blessing* and *anima blessing*. Anthetic Relationship Therapy has found that this meaningful level of interacting is attainable in couples even in conflict. In fact, teaching couples the *animus blessing* and *anima blessing* concept occurs early in the therapeutic process.

The Anthetic terms animus and anima are adaptations of the concepts offered by Jung (Jung, 1961, p. 186). Jung referred to the animus as the unconscious aspects of archetypal masculine properties in a woman's psyche. He labeled the anima as the unconscious archetypal properties in a man's psyche. Jung saw the process of individuation as central to a person's psychological life and posited that making these unconscious elements conscious was essential to individuation. Anthetic Relationship Therapy holds that couples seek both individuation (i.e., greater consciousness) as well as communion (deep, meaningful connecting) through their relationship. To achieve these goals requires skill.

The animus blessing occurs when a man offers a woman words or actions marked by a combination of strength, protection, clarity of understanding, empowerment, and tenderness. Examples occur in ordinary life when a man opens a door for a woman; asks if she needs help with a task; does a task for her; encourages her in doing a task; or teaches her how to actualize her capabilities. The more simple form of blessing, ordinary courtesies, are often conveyed by strangers, yet when given with an attitude of tenderness and caring, produce a psychological impact of profound depth. Some longing in the woman for a masculine blessing, that is, a conferring of a spiritual or deeply meaningful connection with a man occurs. Ideally, the men in a girl's life give the animus blessing throughout her developing years. For example, a daddy refers to his pre-school daughter as "my little princess"; expresses to his pre-teen daughter how much her loves her and assists her with assertive tasks, such as playing sports or riding a bicycle; appreciates his teen daughter in her prom dress ("You'll be the belle of the ball") and accompanies her as she searches for a college to attend. As the daughter receives these blessings, she introjects the approving, loving, appreciating, and empowering messages, thereby internalizing a positive animus in her own psyche. Additionally, girls may receive the animus blessing from brothers, boyfriends, male teachers, coaches, and benevolent strangers.

Once grown, whether having received such blessings or having never received them, the woman longs unconsciously to receive them from her partner. In Anthetic Relationship Therapy, the therapist teaches couples the skill of animus blessing, consisting of seven elements:

1. Behold all parts of the woman from the masculine-as-other perspective. The therapist guides the man to survey his partner's female qualities, traits, characteristics, feelings, and thoughts. Quotes from history or literature can be offered as examples.
2. He pronounces her exquisitely good. Having surveyed her qualities, he now pronounces them exquisitely good. Quotes from history or literature can be offered, as in the excerpt from Harry Truman's letter to Bess: "You know, I've always thought that the best man in the world is hardly good enough for any woman. But when it comes to the best girl in all the universe caring for an ordinary gink like me—well, you'll have to let me get used to it. . . . I've always said I'd have you or no one and that's what I mean to do. . . . I'm all puffed up and hilarious and happy and anything else that happens to a fellow when he finds his lady love thinks more of him than the rest of the beasts" (Geselbracht, 2004).
3. He expresses his male warm approval. The therapist helps him articulate his approval of his partner in warm expressions. For example, "Over all parts of you I cast my strong male look of deep satisfaction and approval" (Elliott, K., & Elliott, J., 2014).
4. He speaks words that cherish. The therapist here guides the man to articulate words of cherishing to his partner. He can in fact use the words, "I cherish you," as well as others that express warmth in this highly valuing way.

5. He assures her of his fidelity. In creating a safe haven, he offers her words that tell of his commitment to always be there for her, for example, "I will never abandon you."
6. He assures her that he will attend to her and give her attention. The therapist helps the man assure that he will attend to not just his partner's profound concerns but also her small qualms and fears. As example, he can offer, "I will be careful to ensure that your slightest fear, your tiniest qualm will get my full care and attention" (Elliott, K., & Elliott, J., 2014). In clinical practice, male partners have exhibited this element in creative ways, including placing a chair in their study and designating it by her name: "This is the Katherine chair."
7. He assures her he blesses her out of free choice and for pleasure. The partner often needs assurance that his blessing is being given freely. The therapist helps the man recognize pleasure in himself at blessing her and helps him speak words of assurance.

Just as the female partner receives the blessing of the masculine from her male partner, so does the male partner thrive when offered the analog, the *anima blessing*. Here the female offers her warm acceptance of what the man gives. She assures him that she warmly receives his blessing and that the impact on her is an increase of her happiness. The anima blessing follows three steps:

1. The female partner increases awareness of the animus blessings the man gives. Here the therapist helps the female partner become aware of ways in which the man has been offering animus blessings about which she may not have been aware.
2. She expresses her receptivity. Having become aware, she now articulates that awareness. Her expressions are warm and honoring.
3. She expresses the positive impact the animus blessing has on her relationship satisfaction. Having recognized the positive impact of the animus blessings she receives, she tenderly expresses the general impact on her happiness and satisfaction in the relationship.

Involvement Skills

Involvement implies more than connection. To be involved is to be caring and to take an interest in the partner's life, interests, and projects. In addition, involvement occurs through curiosity; for example, through Interested Questioning (Chapter 8), together with fully responsive answering. The distinction between connection and involvement is important here. To have a connected conversation means simply to respond directly to what the partner says.

While involvement is first of all a connected response, it also reflects mindfulness of what the speaker is saying and offers an empathic comment based on that mindfulness. Following are examples that clarify the distinctions.

As Jeremy and Amber sit waiting for the arrival of the plane bringing Jeremy's brother for a visit, Jeremy stands up and stretches. Amber asks, "Are you feeling impatient?" Jeremy might respond with a disconnected response: "Planes are always running late." In contrast, connected responses might include, "Yes"; "No"; or "I don't think so." In responding to Amber in an involved way, Jeremy might say, "I might be somewhat impatient. But I'm mostly excited and feeling stiff from sitting so long."

Jeremy's involved response gives respectful consideration to Amber's question and offers substantive information in response. To be involved is to be caring and to offer a fully responsive answer to the partner.

Psychological obstacles partners have evidenced in practicing this skill occur when the partner finds questions such as Amber's painful and hence defend against the pain by withdrawing. Such withdrawal maintains the conversation on a surface level and produces an LVR. For partners who have expressed a desire for greater closeness, the therapist uses the withdrawal as an opportunity to explore the source of the pain, which might include Inner Critic emotional punishments, prototype relationships, or other traumatic interpersonal history.

Empathizing

Empathizing means imagining oneself in the mind of one's partner and seeing things the way he or she does. It includes feeling a partner's feelings as well as thinking a partner's thoughts. Being empathic is vital for creating and sustaining an HVR. Ickes and colleagues (Ickes, 1997; Ickes & Simpson, 1997; Ickes, Stinson, Bissonnette, & Garcia, 1990) offer an expanded definition of empathy labeled *empathic accuracy*; that is, "the degree to which one interactant is able to accurately infer the specific content of another interactant's thoughts and feelings" (p. 731, Ickes, et al., 1990). Research finds that greater empathic accuracy is associated with greater marital satisfaction (Ickes, 1997; Geoff, Fletcher, & Lange, 1997). Moreover, research using physiological measurements of partners' reaction to reliving the other partner's feelings (when watched on videotape) found that when partners relive the other's feelingful experience rather than their own, greater empathy was gauged (Gottman, 1999; Levenson & Ruef, 1992).

Lacking the skill of empathizing will prevent a partner from understanding the motivations behind any of the other partner's requests, thereby creating difficulty in realizing how important they are. In addition, without empathy, when conflicts occur, partners will be unable to see the other's point of view.

Furthermore, when one partner reports feelings of any kind, the other's inability to empathize may lead to discounting those feelings.

Anthetic Relationship Therapy provides the following steps to help partners master the skill of empathizing:

- Step 1: Ask, "Can you tell me more about that?" This question is the first response to a partner reporting a feeling. The listener can ask questions to clarify the other's thoughts and feelings until an accurate understanding of the content occurs. The therapist helps the listener to bracket (i.e., set aside temporarily) his or her own perspective, then imagine being in the other person's mind, seeing his or her reasoning process, in order to imagine how things look from the other person's point of view. Alternatively the partner can use the sentence completion method for more detail. For example, if the partner reports, "I'm worried," the listener can ask, "I'm worried about?" Note that in using this skill, the listener usually begins with the word "I" and speaks as though he or she were the other person.
- Step 2: Eliciting Feelings. If the partner has not reported a feeling but rather an event that is spoken of with a feelingful tone or is *prima facie* an event likely to trigger feelings, the therapist teaches the listener to elicit feelings with the question, "What are you feeling about that?" or "What did you feel when that happened?" For example, if the partner reports, "Our anniversary passed without note again this year," the therapist teaches the listener to ask, "What are you feeling about that?"
- Step 3: Doubling. While the conventional response in the field of therapy is to model and teach reflecting or mirroring feelings (Greenberg & Johnson, 1988), Anthetic Relationship Therapy employs empathic reflection and adds the technique of *empathic doubling*, an adaptation of a method drawn from Psychodrama (Moreno, 1970). The Anthetic adaptation takes the form of a question and always begins with the three words "Is it like?" An example is, "I feel confused about what to do," to which the listener offers the Double: "Is it like 'I've got several options in mind, and I don't know which one is best'?" At this point, the partner responds with either "Yes, yes, that's it" or "No, it's not exactly that; it's more like such-and-such."

Clinical observation has revealed that the empathic double offers a depth of empathy not ordinarily achieved through reflection or empathic mirroring. Couples report that the second person of reflection and mirroring feels more detached and clinical. In contrast, the first person of doubling creates a sense of joining or merging with the other that produces a greater sense of understanding. An additional advantage of doubling is that it is offered through a tentative interrogatory rather than declarative form of mirroring and therefore offers the person who is reporting the feeling an opening to edit more easily.

An important element in empathy between partners is that not only is empathy a responsive skill offered by the listener but also an initiatory skill by the one initiating the report of feelings. When initiating, the skill is termed anticipatory empathy. In this skill, the initiator imagines how the partner might hear what is said and feel in response.

For example, Molly says, "I went with my girlfriend to visit my mother in the hospital, and she said, 'You're looking great!'" In this case, Molly offered an ambiguous antecedent, "she," not clarifying whether the person to whom she referred was her girlfriend or her mother. Using anticipatory empathy, Molly thinks about whether the listener will be able to understand to whom the pronoun refers and edits with, "And my girlfriend said, 'You're looking great!'"

An additional example occurs when a speaker thinks about what feelings a partner might have in hearing what the speaker is saying. Dewey in talking to his wife about the death of one of her three dogs says, "Well, you've still got two more." Dewey has failed to consider how his wife might feel upon hearing his words. The Anthetic Relationship therapist encourages partners to monitor everything they say. With practice, partners find that monitoring becomes automatic and even enjoyable.

Comforting

From time to time, partners may ask to be comforted. Research confirms that couples in the most optimal relationships regularly engage in some form of comforting. The research of Gottman, et al. (1998) found that in happy and stable couples, the wife soothed her husband. (In his research wives used humor.) In Kouneski and Olson's (2004) research, the most intimate and skilled couples were most likely to understand and respond to each other's needs.

In order to increase voltage and engender optimal functioning, Anthetic Relationship Therapy offers couples the skill of comforting. To initiate comforting, the partner must first do Research (Chapter 12) about what form of comforting is being requested. Clinical experience indicates that partners find various expressions comforting; for some it is touch, while for others it is words of soothing.

When partners find it difficult to provide comforting, the therapist may facilitate exploration, either through sentence stem completion or through Anthetic Dialogue to discover Inner Critic shoulds that pejoratize comforting as "weakness" or "softness." Once such a should is revealed, the therapist can assist the person in challenging the Inner Critic; for example, "I have the right to ask for comforting" or "I have the right to give comforting."

Expressing Positivity

While researchers found that positivity is essential in not only preventing divorce but also creating optimal functioning in marriages, they also discovered that simply exhorting a couple to be more positive or even declaring love days is insufficient for helping a couple increase positivity (Gottman, 1999). One key problem to the puzzling failure of attempts by therapists to increase positivity in order to produce more marital stability was the finding that only happy couples (not unhappy ones) were enhanced through positivity. In unhappy marriages, positivity became fodder in the mill of the climate of negative perception of the partners.

Anthetic Relationship Therapy holds that positivity is essential for producing optimality when it is targeted (i.e., specific to the partner) and when it is focused on elements about which the partner values being seen. Expressing positivity emerges out of partners' beholding of each other followed by communication of the impact of the beholding.

Expressing positivity includes giving praise, appreciations, likings, and admiration. Following are examples:

- "I like it when you. . ."
- "What I appreciate about you is. . ."
- "What I like about you is. . ."
- "You're special because. . ."
- "You're important to me because. . ."
- "You're a good friend to me because. . ."
- "I really admire your. . ."
- "Thanks for being so. . ."
- "You're a remarkable person because of your. . ."
- "You're very skilled at. . ."

Each of the above, when the sentence is completed, is a positive stroke. They are part of the glue that holds HVRs together.

One caution about which the therapist may warn couples is not to give global praise, which can lead to interchanges such as the following:

"I think you're wonderful!"
"Oh? What is wonderful about me?"
"Everything!"
"Can you be specific?"
"No. It's *everything!*"

The positive strokes contained in the Positivity skills are based on mindfulness of the partner's good points. It requires a movement out of self-centeredness on the part of the one expressing positivity; thinking about the partner in detail and seeing in depth their assets.

In clinical experience, a number of psychological obstacles have emerged in partners learning this skill. Many partners enter marriage with childhood learning not to give positive strokes. Typical comments are "It's silly," "He or she doesn't need my praise," and "I don't want to give him/her a swelled head." Having never seen positivity modeled in family of origin interactions, partners lack awareness that it is technically possible to give many positive strokes per day. Primary in the educational tasks of therapy is to provide couples with the knowledge and skill that positivity can be a part of daily life for the couple.

Other blocks that have emerged in clinical couple work is based on polar type rigidity. For example, Tough Self-Sufficient partners often protest, "Why should I praise someone for doing what they're supposed to do anyway?" Contained in such a question are implicit shoulds to not need anyone and to not "baby" anyone or "be babied."

Still another block revealed in processing work is the belief that praising another implies that the one giving praise is inferior. This belief is the result of Inner Critic messages that fuse praising another with being one-down.

Not only is the giving of positivity important, but also essential is the response of the person receiving the positive communication. Reciprocal positive responses include a simple statement of gratitude ("Thank you"); a self-disclosure of the impact of the positive comment (i.e., "That feels so good"); and an agreement with the comment ("Yes, I thought so too").

While positivity is an important need for most humans, a number of psychological barriers may emerge in therapy as the couple practice the positivity skill. One such barrier is giving a deflecting response (i.e., "Well, I had a lot of help"). Such a response emerges when Inner Critic messages in the recipient include condemnation that to accept positivity is to be egotistical. Once revealed in therapy and labeled as an Inner Critic message, the therapist can help the person use the "What You Call Technique" for challenging (Elliott, J., & Elliott, K., 2000, p. 138) by saying to the Inner Critic, "I have the right to be what you call egotistical."

Another frequent barrier to positivity noted in research occurs when a couple exhibits a pattern of negative attributions for even positive partner behaviors (Berley & Jacobson, 1984; Gottman, 1999; Watzlawick, Beavin, & Jackson (1967). In such cases, Anthetic Relationship Therapy for reducing negativity (Chapter 9) precedes positivity skills.

In summary, an essential ingredient in creating an optimally functioning

HVR is generous praise throughout the day given by both partners. Therapy in which negativity reduction skills are followed by positivity skills equips the couple to create a climate of optimality.

Celebratory Skills

An important element of positivity is the practice of celebratory skills. When a partner reports a pleasurable experience or a triumph, whether major or minor, the other partner gives positive strokes to help the person celebrate the occasion. Clinical experience indicates that genuine celebration of each other's pleasures and triumphs supports intimacy; that is, "the extent to which the partners share knowledge regarding each other's personally meaningful and emotionally charged experiences." (Ickes, Hutchison, & Mashek, 2004, p. 358).

Examples of celebratory communications include:

- "Wow!"
- "That's wonderful!"
- "Good for you!"
- "You must be feeling great!"
- "I'm so happy for you!"
- "Tell me the details."

A prerequisite for expressing celebration is the ability to empathize. Empathy creates an experience of shared joy. If either partner has a block to empathizing, the therapist must turn to teaching the skill of empathizing mentioned earlier in this chapter.

Giving "Thank You's"

While saying, "Thank You" is an element in common courtesy, doing so also can be an important element in creating an optimal relationship. It becomes so when "Thank you" statements are an expression of an attitude of gratitude of one partner toward another. As one partner behaves in a way that is helpful, kind, or loving, and the other partner responds with gratitude, a climate of generosity emerges. Such a climate, researchers note, is positively associated with marital satisfaction (Dew & Wilcox, 2013).

Chapter 11

Handling the Voltage Mismatch

Because high-voltage relating seems prima facie so desirable in terms of its ability to fulfill needs for closeness and intimacy, one would think that everyone would desire it. However, not only has clinical experience revealed that this is not true but also social psychology research has affirmed it. Intimate relationships are predicated upon intersubjectivity; that is, two persons share a common perspective of the nature of their relationship (Ickes, Hutchison, & Mashek, 2004). Moreover, in order to relate in a high-voltage way, partners engage in what Crossley (1996) called radical intersubjectivity. In this mode of relating, two people transcend subjective perspectives into a "common ground"; a "common world" (Crossley, 1996, p. 33). They merge with each other as found in A. Aron and his colleagues' self-expansion research, in such a way that boundaries between self and other dissolve and interdependence intensifies (Aron, A., & Aron, E.N., 1997; Aron, A., Aron, E.N., & Smollan, 1992).

The ability to engage in this type of intense intimacy is not universal. Research on modes of social relating has revealed that an entire group of research subjects who were involved in close relationships were averse to closeness (Mashek & Sherman, 2004). The individuals in this group shunned closeness and preferred distance even in their intimate relationships. Compared to others in the study, individuals in this group were less likely to desire affection; less likely to want to know their partner in-depth; more likely to feel humiliated; and more likely to experience self-hatred. They reported a greater propensity for feeling suffocated and smothered in their relationships, which they characterized as "too close." From an attachment model perspective, this group fit the profile of those who are avoidant in attachment style. Using the Anthetic Voltage model, this group corresponds to low-voltage functioning.

Low-voltage (closeness-averse; avoidant) functioning serves as a coping strategy in the face of perceived threats. This strategy becomes problematic in romantic relationships, as seen in research studying avoidant individuals' ability to provide support when their partners are in need of it. In one study (Fraley & Shaver, 1998), when partners were about to part at an airport due to travel, the avoidant partner was less likely to provide caregiving behaviors to his or her partner upon parting. In another study by Simpson, Rholes, & Nelligan (1992), females in heterosexual romantic relationships were told they were facing a painful, anxiety-provoking situation. In response, when females were more distressed, their avoidant male partners were less supportive. A summary of findings in such studies suggests that avoidant partners may be unsupportive and distant during situations where partners would likely need support. Also at those times, avoidant partners are more likely to be unresponsive and avoid communication regarding emotion-laden issues (B.C. Feeney & Collins, 2001; Fraley & Shaver, 1998; Simpson et al., 1992; Collins & B.C. Feeney, 2000; Simpson, Rholes, & Phillips, 1996). Over time, avoidant individuals' pattern of distancing themselves, non-communicating, and suppressing negative emotion often leads to relationship dissatisfaction, deterioration, and dissolution (Edelstein & Shaver, 2004). For the partner of an avoidant person, the net result is a great deal of emotional pain and damage.

Moreover, a voltage mismatch, that is, when one partner is high voltage and the other functions in a low-voltage way, will produce pain for *each* partner. The high-voltage partner will feel the pain of being abandoned and ignored. The low-voltage partner will feel the pain of being suffocated and tormented. The result will be the Pursuer-Distancer pattern, the desperate Pursuer and the equally desperate Distancer, each trying to legislate a special agenda through anger and judgmentalism. The result is a great many ferocious arguments that may ultimately tear the couple apart. Therefore, an important purpose in addressing the mismatch may be to save the relationship.

The voltage mismatch is a common profile presented by couples in therapy. One impetus for the couple to seek therapy is an interesting occurrence reported to Anthetic relationship therapists called the *whiff.* A whiff occurs when a high-voltage partner experiences a sample of what a HVR would be like. Following are examples reported by clients in therapy:

- Lynn attended a teachers' convention. While waiting for an elevator, a man spoke kindly to her. She was astonished and overcome with emotion. The kindness was in stark contrast to her husband's communications to her that were consistently critical, contemptuous, and gruff. By experiencing this simple act, Lynn was able to tell herself, "So this is what it's like to be the recipient of kindness." She had experienced a whiff. She returned home and stated an ultimatum to her husband: "Either you come with me to therapy or I'm moving out."

- Maryetta was a full-time homemaker and mother. One day a carpenter came to install kitchen cabinets in her home, and she began talking with him. In fact, she poured out her heart to him. He listened with great empathy and gentleness. This was also a "whiff" situation. For the first time in years, she experienced the feeling of having someone listen deeply to her.
- Bob kept to himself at work but one day found himself sitting next to a female co-worker in the company cafeteria on their coffee break. "She didn't speak harshly to me about anything!" he said. "I got a whiff of what it was like to be with a woman who simply had good will toward me."
- Andrew was on a flight for business and was seated behind a couple who were mature in age. They sat with their heads together talking intimately. Andrew reported that at that moment, he realized that what the couple shared, he did not have with his wife but keenly desired. Upon returning home from the trip, he told his wife of the whiff and requested she attend counseling with him in order to learn to achieve what he had witnessed in the couple.

Often paired with the whiff experience is another realization that is called an *awakening*. It is as though the person has been sleepwalking but wakes up to see things from a new perspective. Behavior the partner had been thinking of as normal now seems "not quite right" or even "terribly wrong." Following are examples reported in therapy:

- Negativity (emotional abuse) no longer seems acceptable. The partner is no longer willing to simply overlook it. He or she now demands respect.
- When irrationality happens, it now becomes clear. For example, the partner says, "I'm always wrong!" When the other says, "No you're not; you were right in what you said this morning," the partner's response of "See? Wrong again!" becomes clear as a case of irrationality and a no-win situation.
- In a case where a person has been waiting on the partner who is participating in infidelity to decide between the spouse and the lover, his or her previous position had been, "If you can't choose between me and someone else, I'll just wait until you make up your mind, no matter how long it takes." After the whiff experience, an awakening occurs and the partner's new perspective is, "What in the world have I been thinking, to wait until someone makes a decision about me? If he can't decide, I'm not staying."
- A person may have an existential awakening, as in the case of Marilyn, whose aunt died. Marilyn suddenly became aware of the brevity of life. "Death is going to happen to me, too," she thought. "Am I going to keep putting up with my unhappy relationship until I die?" She sought counseling and began making changes in her life.

Other awakenings occur when a "model"; someone who is proactively having a fulfilling and satisfying relationship, inspires possibilities for personal satisfaction in the observer. In addition, advice received from a friend, a therapist, or a book to leave a destructive relationship may be one more factor in a partner's re-assessment.

Shortly after the whiff experience and the awakening experience, the person typically engages in a re-assessment of the relationship in which he or she is living. Variations of such a person's re-evaluative thoughts include, "What am I doing in a relationship where I'm not valued and respected?" or "Why am I valuing someone who doesn't value me?" or "I'm suddenly realizing my partner values me for the wrong reasons."

Confronting the Mismatch: The Three Options

When couples present in therapy, they have frequently been motivated to do so out of some progression through the whiff, the awakening, and a re-assessment. Despite their emerging awareness of a problem in the relationship sufficiently severe to seek therapy, partners in a relationship pattern consistent with a voltage mismatch are usually puzzled as to the unhappiness they are experiencing. As the therapist listens to a description of their difficulties, a case conceptualization evolves in which the partners' Pursuer-Distancer style is suggestive of a voltage disparity. The therapist may then offer a voltage questionnaire, such as the Checklist in Chapter 1. Partners may discuss their answers and self-assess their voltage desires. When a couple realizes their difficulties have their origins in a voltage disparity, the therapist can offer three options for proceeding.

Option one consists of a decision on the part of the high-voltage person to increase his or her tolerance for the low-voltage style of the partner. This shift can occur by the high-voltage partner lowering expectations and learning skills for adjusting to an LVR. The person may develop interests that decrease the high-voltage partner's dependency on the low-voltage partner for need gratification.

Option two involves a decision by the low-voltage partner to engage in therapeutic work to increase tolerance for high-voltage by learning high-voltage skills.

Option three occurs when partners decide to terminate the relationship. In clinical experience, partners usually attempt options one or two prior to choosing option three. However, the writers have seen partners choose option three when the relationship is not one involving marital commitment, where no children are involved, and where emotional attachment to each other was minimal or so eroded that attending therapy was a final step in a process of dissolution that was already well underway.

Research findings regarding the preferability of the first two options offer important considerations for guiding couples in differential decision making. Choosing either of options one or two in order to continue the relationship can produce what Gottman (1999, p. 95) called perpetual problems. In his study of partners who were mismatched in conflict resolution styles, that is, in emotional expressiveness and influence functions, even when able to make adjustments to an "in-between" type, continued to have ongoing conflict, pain, and feelings of rejection regarding differences in the amount of deep connection they wanted. Frequently, partners in Anthetic Relationship Therapy ask whether they can achieve medium voltage. Gottman's research seems to imply a Yes answer, with the caveat that the couple attempting to do so can expect a predictable cost in terms of satisfaction and lack of optimality.

The Anthetic Relationship Therapy approach has as its goal optimality and encourages couples to learn the high-voltage skills needed for optimal satisfaction. However, choice among the three options is the decision of the couple. If the couple choose to engage in the change process toward high voltage, both partners inevitably ask, "Can a person change from low-voltage to high-voltage?" This question echoes an ongoing one in relationship literature regarding whether a person can change when he or she exhibits an avoidant attachment style, feelings of self-hatred, and a self-sufficient pattern of functioning. Because of their dislike of self-disclosure, along with their avoidance of addressing needs in themselves and others, such individuals are particularly difficult to treat in therapy (Edelstein & Shaver, 2004).

Nevertheless, progress in the field of relationship therapy is occurring in treatment of individuals who exhibit avoidant, self-sufficient, and defensive styles. Contributions to treatment have been made by Firestone and Catlett (1999) who address "the Voice," the internalized negative messages occurring in partners and leading to defensiveness and conflict. Another approach is Emotionally Focused Therapy (Johnson, 1996), which helps partners who bring an attachment wound to their adult relationships to use one another as sources of comfort, thus producing a secure attachment bond. In addition, object-relations therapists (Scharff & Scharff, 1987) help couples gain insight into origins of their defensive strategies, thus reducing projection of negative introjected objects onto one another.

Understanding the Psychodyanamics of Low-Voltage

In order to understand some of the difficulty entailed in change in a person with a low-voltage style, it is essential to understand the subconscious dynamics that fuel it. The high-voltage partner often has the illusion that conversion to high-voltage functioning is a simple matter, like teaching someone to enjoy good music. What the high-voltage person finds so difficult to understand is that the low-voltage person is secretly terrified. Powerful subconscious forces in the low-voltage person prevent him or her from even considering a high-voltage way of relating. For example, the low-voltage person has powerful Inner Critic shoulds not to be seen as weak or vulnerable. Before any change can possibly take place, those forces must be surfaced, identified, and neutralized, a process that is done in Anthetic Relationship Therapy sessions. In addition, the low-voltage person has learned to associate closeness with attachment injury or other interpersonal pain carried from childhood. Because low-voltage functioning is a defense against the resurfacing of that pain, heavy pressure from the partner or the therapist can lead to decompensation, accompanied by an intense Inner Critic attack, and occurrence of depression or anxiety. It therefore is imperative that the therapist's strategy must be (a) to move slowly; (b) to make sure the low-voltage person accepts and owns the Anthetic values; (c) to assure the low-voltage person that the therapist and partner understand how difficult this process is; and (d) to provide large amounts of soothing and praise throughout the process.

The Protocol for Changing from Low-Voltage to High-Voltage

Whether a person is low voltage and wants to change or high voltage and wants to better handle the voltage, Anthetic Relationship Therapy offers the following protocol. In this process, the therapist guides the person in making the necessary values choices, learning foundational concepts, gaining skills, and engaging in interpersonal processes that foster high-voltage functioning. All of these elements are the focus of this book. The following protocol serves as a meta-guide for proceeding:

1. Make a Value Shift. The therapist helps the person shift from valuing the protection of being low voltage to the riskiness of being high voltage. The shift must take place on the basis of faith that the high-voltage position will, in the long run, result in more satisfaction that the low-voltage position. (See Chapter 5 for guidance in values choice work.)
2. Read *Disarming Your Inner Critic* (Elliott, J., & Elliott, K., 2000). Because the Inner Critic is the primary psychodynamic source of the low-voltage defense structure, it is essential that the person understands its functioning in his or her life and learn skills for becoming free from its influence. The *Disarming* book, written for consumers as well as professionals, has been used with clients in therapy with great success.
3. Practice Self-Monitoring. The therapist guides the person to think before he or she talks, for example, when about to make a factual statement, to

evaluate it for accuracy before saying it. If about to say something about his or her partner, the therapist teaches to ask himself or herself whether the statement will be angry or judgmental. If it is, the person is guided not to act it out, but rather to report it as a pull; for example, "I have a pull to see you as a bad person, but I'm not going to go there."

4. Become proficient in making Anthetic releasing statements. This step is essential in order to handle the high-voltage of feedback. Releasing statements are described in great detail in *Disarming Your Inner Critic*.
5. Request feedback from one's partner about whatever task on which one is working. For example, if a partner is working on reducing negativity or distancing, this feedback is crucial, since people usually are not aware of what they are doing. The form for requesting can be, "I have a request you tell me whenever you see me distancing by asking, 'Are you feeling distant?' or 'You seem distant.'" Upon receiving the feedback, the recipient can say, "Thank you for telling me."
6. Request general feedback from one's partner on progress being made in moving from low voltage to high voltage. Clinical experience indicates progress is maximized when asking for general feedback occurs at a minimum of two or three times a week. In addition, asking for feedback in terms of a report card grade from "A" to "F" is helpful.
7. When receiving disconfirmatory feedback, make one or more Anthetic releasing statements. Hearing a lower grade than expected can trigger Inner Critic emotional pain. Any negative emotions can be handled by identifying the Inner Critic should that was triggered and then using a releasing statement to get free from the emotional pain. The skill of making releasing statements is absolutely essential for having a successful HVR. The therapist reframes disconfirmatory feedback (that disconfirms one's self-image) by explaining that it is not criticism, but rather is valuable information. It may feel like harsh criticism unless the person can learn to make releasing statements, whereupon it is transformed into growth-centered feedback.

   For example, the person may be told by her partner, "What you just said sounded judgmental." This is a high-voltage statement that requires the wiring to handle it and use it toward growth. The metaphor of the electrician is often helpful to offer: "Consider the electrician who works on a job, touching live wires here and there without rubber gloves and other protective gear. The power is high and chances are she'll get burned. The releasing statements are your rubber gloves. If you try to have a high-voltage relationship without having learned the protective skills afforded by the releasing statements, you'll feel burned too. You may even feel attacked; figuratively beaten up. It will look as though it's the doing of your partner, but it will really be the doing of your Inner Critic. In order to learn to use the 'rubber gloves' of releasing statements, use the *Disarming* book, which may be all you'll need or we can work on them in a session."

Two additional metaphors that have helped partners in therapy reframe feedback as beneficial is by comparing feedback regarding relationship functioning as akin to feedback from a tennis coach and as comparable to feedback given in Toastmasters.

8. Ask the therapist about anything not understood. The therapist must encourage the person to ask questions, especially for help in making releasing statements.
9. Keep a notebook. A notebook is beneficial to the change process in several ways: It is a useful record of insights gained, analyses of arguments, concepts and skills learned, and handouts received. For example, an analysis of an argument might answer the following questions: How did the argument start? What triggered my stuff? What shoulds were involved? What buffers were threatened? Was I in an Inner Figure? Did I use releasing statements? Or did I try to get acquitted? How did the argument get resolved? The therapist encourages the partners to read the notebook at least once a day and to discuss it with each other.
10. Meditate often on a "hot list" selected from one's notebook. This list can be written on a 4x6 card, which can be kept with the person at all times and consulted often. It should consist of approximately a dozen brief items the person would like to keep in mind. The person should read this "litany," or hot list, out loud to the partner three or four times a day.
11. Make a recording based on the hot list. The therapist encourages the person to listen to the recording every morning and evening.
12. Whenever the partners begin an argument, stop talking, come to a halt, listen to the recording and read the notes in the notebook. This requires that the person bracket any pride and expose himself or herself to the new learning contained in the material.
13. Attend Anthetic Relationship Therapy frequently. It is recommended that partners in change attend therapy a minimum of once a week and at first more frequently.
14. Discuss progress with one's partner. The therapist recommends that at least once a day but preferably two or three times a day partners discuss their progress with one another. The first topic should be the results of meditation on one's process.
15. Take the work seriously. Partners may defend against the intensity by using humor. However, the therapist should warn partners about this defense and recommend they maintain a serious attitude to the change process.

Dealing with Resistance

The structures of low-voltage relating are rooted in ingrained and highly valued strategies for protection from pain and for feelings of self-esteem. Resistance to change will frequently occur in partners for a number of reasons listed below. Experimental research indicates that avoidant people (those who fit what in the voltage model is described as low voltage) respond positively to security inducing primes, becoming less hostile, more empathic, and more attracted to secure relationship partners (Baldwin, Keelan, Fehr, Enns, & Koh-Rangarajoo, 1996; Edelstein & Shaver, 2004; Mikulincer & Shaver, 2001; Mikulincer et al., 2001). Guided by this research, therapeutic interventions that enhance security are essential. Therefore the voltage change process in each of the following examples of resistance involves guiding the higher voltage partner to use the skill of listening for Laments paired with giving the anthetic sacrament.

1. The high-voltage partner may have been expressing anger and judgmentalism toward the low-voltage partner in an attempt to pressure him or her to change. In response, the low-voltage partner becomes more distant, often saying, "I'm distancing because I can't take your fussing at me anymore. It's too painful." If this is the case, the therapist must help the high-voltage person work on his or her judgmentalism in order to reduce it. This will involve identifying Inner Critic and other Inner Figure elements and learning to disengage from them.
2. The low-voltage partner fears being hurt. In childhood, the low-voltage person was a prospective high-voltage person. However, he or she usually became traumatized, often by parents, but sometimes in a romantic relationship. Because of the dysfunctional learning taken from the trauma, the incipient high-voltage person then made an early decision: "From now on I'm never going to get hurt again. I'll be Tough or Self-Sufficient or both. Nobody is ever going to get close to me. It's too painful."
3. The low-voltage individual fears being seen and known. This can be traced to a strong Inner Critic that tells the low-voltage person that their thoughts, feelings, and personal qualities are defective. To expose them would be humiliating. Therefore, the low-voltage person develops guardedness and withdrawal as a defense against potential Inner Critic condemnation consisting of "You're defective"; "You're inferior"; or "You're guilty." The distancing solution, while a relief for the low-voltage person is a source of pain to the high-voltage partner.
4. The low-voltage person fears what other people might think if he or she loses some of the Toughness and Self-Sufficiency of the defense structure and becomes Tender and Dependent. People might think he or she was weak or defective.

5. The low-voltage person fears having a successful relationship. In clinical experience, a not uncommon fear is feeling guilty by surpassing Mom and Dad in this respect.
6. The low-voltage person fears putting his or her partner first, because that means rejecting someone else. In cases of poor individuation, the person fears that putting his or her partner first will trigger the Inner Critic pleading him or her guilty of the crime of being disloyal to children, parents, or friends.
7. The low-voltage person fears growing up and becoming an adult. Although growing up engenders a feeling of freedom, low-voltage persons may feel burdened by having to learn the required skills. They additionally may feel hemmed in, which because of their self-sufficiency is aversive.
8. The low-voltage person fears that high-voltage functioning would result in the loss of a melodramatic style in which he or she was living. The melodramatic style holds value because it is counter-depressive.
9. The low-voltage person fears closeness in which he or she would be seen as "not good enough." This fear has its source in a should to be perfect, rather than human.
10. The low-voltage person believes that successful relating depends not on sharing the anthetic values (Chapter 5) but only on giving material things such as money or expensive gifts to his or her partner.
11. The low-voltage person has such a strong need to feel superior that he or she resists giving up the safety of this position. The strength of this need lies in the compensatory value of feeling superior in defending against Inner Critic condemnation.

Two Cases

When first presented with the concept of HV and LV relationships, many clients in couple therapy become fascinated. Some realize that high voltage is what they have always wanted but for which they did not have a concept. In addition, with the application of the low-voltage and high-voltage categories, many puzzling elements in their relationships suddenly begin to be understandable. Many see that they had been high-voltage people in relationships with low-voltage partners experiencing all the conflict and dissatisfaction of the voltage mismatch. Once presented with the options for dealing with the mismatch, many choose Option two, seeking to change the low-voltage partner into high voltage. In order to equip therapists to distinguish outcome in such therapeutic endeavors, the following two case histories of change attempts are offered, one unsuccessful and the other successful.

The first case concerns Todd and Marissa, an unsuccessful change process. Todd was 40, a successful stockbroker. Marissa was 33, an illustrator. The couple had no children. As a high-voltage person she thought it normal for men to be distant. She tried to adjust to the distance in their relationship but failed. To her surprise, Todd came with her to therapy but only as an observer. Todd thought their marriage was great. He based his assessment on their possessions: an expensive house, two late-model cars, European vacations. He was puzzled at Marissa's dissatisfaction. She, in turn, thought there was probably something wrong with her and wondered if she was having a mid-life crisis.

In therapy, Marissa began to voice some complaints. She wanted more affection, deeper involvement, and more communication. Todd did not understand the depth of her pain and did not take her requests seriously.

Marissa: I wanted him to bring me flowers, but he wouldn't. I finally nagged him into doing it, so one day he came home, threw some roses on the table, and said, 'Here's your damned flowers!' I cried the rest of the night. He still thinks flowers are unimportant. 'They just die after a while,' he says.

Then I hinted about more affection. When that didn't work, I made requests. Then he got really angry. I told him I was thinking of leaving him. He just dismissed my complaints. He had talked to his friends about the situation, and they said, 'She'll get over it. She doesn't really mean she'd leave you over a little thing like that. She's just grouchy. Maybe it's that time of the month.'

He won't take me seriously. And then I left him. He kept calling and pleading with me to come back. He said, 'Let's put this behind us and start over,' but I knew that wouldn't work. He's got to make some changes in himself.

Todd: That would be pretty private. Even if I do get in therapy, you can't expect me to report like a criminal to his probation officer. That's right isn't it?

Therapist: Well, it sounds like that's what Marissa wants. And if you feel like a criminal, that's your Inner Critic talking. If you choose to give her what she wants, I can help you with that.

Marissa: That's exactly what I want. I've got to know what's going on with you so I can tell whether I want to continue this relationship.

Todd: Well, it's like you're testing me. That's no good. I don't like being tested.

Marissa: (Thoughtful) Yes, I guess that is exactly what I'm doing: testing you. I don't mind being tested, and I don't want someone as a partner who doesn't welcome it with open arms. It's as simple as that.

Without reply, Todd stood up and stalked out of the consulting room, slamming the door. Marissa spent the rest of the session talking about the possibility of divorce. She attended a few more sessions, as the divorce proceeded, and then reported that she had met a man who was compatible with her in functioning in a high-voltage way.

Marissa: I don't know whether I'm ready for a new relationship so soon, but it's nice to know there are men out there who are like me. Todd was like my dad, cool and distant. Being with my new friend is scary, because I'm not sure I have anything to give him, but I'm willing to handle the scariness with him instead of the pain I was feeling with Todd.

She returned six months later, reporting that her divorce had become final and that she felt more happiness that she had ever felt in her life. While this case is being reported as unsuccessful, for Marissa it was a success.

The following case involves a successful change from low voltage to high voltage. Benjamin, who functioned as a Self-Sufficient low-voltage person, had always had great difficulty with relationships. Benjamin's wife, Marianna, reported that she could sense just under the layer of Self-Sufficiency a tremendous need for love, a deep hunger.

Marianna had threatened to leave Benjamin if he did not become more affectionate, and Benjamin was feeling some pain about that. The pain was sufficient to motivate him to work toward change. He was also puzzled by his previous relationship failures, and he was willing to take a risk and try something new. Benjamin's relationship history is consistent with research findings regarding avoidant, self-sufficient individuals, suggesting that their romantic relationships are characterized by lower levels of satisfaction, intimacy, and longevity (Brennan & Shaver, 1995; B.C. Feeney & Collns, 2001; J.A. Feeney, 1998, 1999; Kirkpatrick & David, 1994; Kirkpatrick & Hazan, 1994; Lussier, Sabourin, & Turgeon, 1997).

The first goal of Anthetic Relationship Therapy with this couple was to help Marianna process and reduce her judgmentalism. The therapist helped her soften her heart and express love in a one-way fashion, not expecting reciprocity. Marianna also learned to recognize Benjamin's laments and to give him the deep empathy of the anthetic sacrament.

The therapist began work with Benjamin by teaching him to challenge the following commands issued by his Inner Critic: "Be self-sufficient. Don't get close. Be a Lone Wolfe; otherwise, you'll get hurt again."

Therapist: Your task is to learn how to melt your heart and become like a playful puppy-dog; like Odie in the *Garfield* comic strip.

Benjamin: (Grimacing) But I don't want to be mushy!

Therapist: That's exactly what I want to do to help you improve your relationship with Marianna. I want to give you "mushiness lessons."

Benjamin: (Laughs)

The therapist noted mentally that Benjamin's inner figure, a Playful Child, had been the one to laugh, both intrigued and fascinated. Benjamin had difficulty making releasing statements, at first not understanding the concept of getting released. However, suddenly, as frequently happens, he comprehended it. As he made the releasing statements, he took back his right to be mushy and to be feminine (which he had equated with being tender).

In addition, Benjamin read *Disarming Your Inner Critic*, and then re-read it. He made a project of continual re-reading, each time making new notes in the margins. He created a litany card, which he reviewed and spoke to Marianna frequently: "I value closeness, not distance. I value pleasure, not revenge. I prioritize getting disconfirming feedback over avoiding humiliation. I make releasing statements whenever I hear such feedback." This litany established the values shift Benjamin was choosing to make. By declaring them out loud to Marianna, he not only strengthened his Executive Self, he also communicated to Marianna an important statement of the kind of relationship he wanted. He was well on the way to softening his heart and learning to handle high voltage. His intrapsychic work toward the goal of an HVR was successful.

The problem to address then remained Marianna's impulses to be judgmental. Once she had made a value shift from revenge to closeness, the work she did was effective. She saw how her judgmentalism served as a buffer, and she resolved to seek self-esteem in other ways, primarily by challenging her Inner Critic messages and becoming free. Benjamin gave her feedback every time he spotted her judgmentalism, which she welcomed with a releasing statement, followed by Researching and other feedback processing steps.

With intrapsychic skills in place, the therapist then began to teach the couple the interpersonal skills for high-voltage relating (Chapters 8 and 9). The couple reported enjoying a satisfying HVR.

In reviewing the distinction between cases that are successful and those that are not, one important factor emerges. The more fused the person is with the low-voltage defense structure, the poorer prognosis for change. The greater access to the Black Hole, that is, a yearning for closeness, the more positive prognosis. The more fully the partners, both low-voltage and high-voltage take responsibility for personal change, the better the prognosis. In any case, upon the partners' request for change, the therapist offers as much of the model's approach as partners can withstand, whether values, intrapsychic skills, or interpersonal skills.

Chapter 12

Maintenance Skills

High Voltage for a Lifetime

As mentioned in Chapter 1, humans are made for romantic love (Aron, Fisher, Mashek, Strong, Haifang, & Brown, 2005). Moreover, contrary to previous conventional and professional theory, research now shows that the intense euphoria of early stage romantic love can continue for a lifetime (Aron, et al., 2005).

The field of relationship science is providing marital therapists a body of research upon which to build clinical interventions for greater closeness and intimacy in personal relationships (see Duck, 1997; Fletcher & Clark, 2000; Kelley, Berscheid, Christensen, Harvey, Huston, Levinger, 1983; and Mashek & Aron, 2004 for compendia of findings).

The HVR model equips couples not only to achieve optimal closeness in the initial stages of an intimate relationship, but it also articulates strategies for maintaining optimality for a lifetime. This chapter will provide concepts and skills for doing so.

Checking Skills

The high-voltage climate is predicated upon self-disclosure, forthcomingness, and ongoing communication as to the state of the relationship. Equipped with *checking skills*, partners can stay in close connection, gleaning information from each other, and attending to the needs of each other and the relationship.

The first skill is checking for communication effectiveness. As a speaker each partner checks intermittently to determine whether he or she has been communicating effectively. To do this, the partner asks for feedback from the listener. While there are many ways to do this, two examples are:

- "Is it clear what I'm saying?"
- "Did I answer your question?"

The second checking skill involves checking for love or liking. In order to maintain an HVR it is necessary that partners ask each other for reports of love or liking. The checking statement consists of two questions. First, is "Do you love me?" (or "Do you like me?"). The partners also, after an argument ask, "Do you still love me?"

Examples of possible connected answers include, "Yes," "Sometimes," or "No." Examples of disconnected answers include, "That's a silly question"; "I wouldn't be here if I didn't love/like you"; "You are loved; don't you believe it?" or "You sound pretty insecure."

The question is more than a request for information. It is a request for the expression of liking, or love, or perhaps warm feelings. A partner's disinterest in expressing such feelings is indicative of a lack of interest in a HVR.

The second question asked upon receiving a "Yes" to the first questions is "What do you like (or love) about me?" While a common answer from partners is "I love *everything* about you," such a global response will not bring the couple closer. The therapist's task is then teaching the responding partner to offer details regarding elements he or she values. Partners frequently find it helpful to consider categories of characteristics (e.g., physical, emotional, relational, intellectual, spiritual) in order to kindle the response process.

The third checking skill involves researching. Researching is one variety of Interested Questioning and is the opposite of defending and controlling. It is essential in checking out assumptions a person might be making about something his or her partner thinks or feels. For example, Clay said in a couple session, "I don't have to ask my wife. I know she hates honesty." When the therapist suggested he research his assumption with his wife, Narya, she said, "No, that's how I used to be. Now I want honesty."

A Researching communication can be either initiatory or responsive. An example of an initiatory research question would be, "I think you would prefer to stay home tonight, is that right?" Another example would be, "I noticed you had a change of expression when I told you about running into my old girlfriend today. I think you felt scared, is that right?"

A responsive research question is used when a partner has disclosed a thought or feeling, such as, "I'd like us to move to a new house." The research question would be, "Tell me more about that."

Hyperbolic Expressiveness

While almost tacitly obvious, research also supports that positive expressions of love and affection are associated with greater satisfaction in marriages (Weiss, 1980; Gottman, 1999). For the maintenance of high-voltage relating for a lifetime, couples are encouraged to engage in *hyperbolic expressiveness*. The term is defined as expressions of love, affection, and beholding in extravagant dimensions. The therapist encourages the couple to engage in writing love notes, reading love poems to one another, singing love songs, and surrounding themselves with images of love and romance. The content of such communications is extravagant, as in "I love you more than life itself" and "I hold you way above all other women (or men)."

The Anthetic Dialogue of Ideas

Not infrequently couples in therapy state, "Oh, that's a hot topic. We learned long ago we just can't go there." Statements such as this represent an attempt to manage differences in ideas and the anxiety they trigger by agreeing on cells of topics that are taboo. Unfortunately, such albeit agreed-upon injunctions against talking produce a diminishment of closeness. Neither partner knows what the other is thinking, and opportunities for mutual enrichment are lost. The high-voltage model offers the *Anthetic Dialogue of Ideas* process to provide partners optimal satisfaction for the exchange of ideas. The process is based on the following principles:

1. Each person maintains an open mind and is receptive to being influenced by the other.
2. Each person holds his or her position as provisional, that is, not absolutely certain. The provisionality must be indicated by such a statement as, "I may be wrong, but here's my opinion."
3. The provisionality is also indicated by such statements as, "Let me think about that. Hmmm." Kneejerk reactions are prohibited.
4. Since reactive attachment to ideas will prevent partners from carefully considering opposing points of view, each must disengage from any attachment and switch into considering any assertion as a hypothesis, not a certain "fact." This switch will permit each to use the provisional style that is necessary for the Anthetic Dialogue of Ideas.
5. It is incumbent on the person presenting an assertion to be prepared to offer adequate support for its validation. This support may consist of evidence or other reasons for believing the assertion. No unsupported assertions are permitted. The request for such support may be made by asking questions such as "How do you know that?" "What reasons can you offer for believing that?" and "Why do you think that's a valid statement?"
6. Each partner must enthusiastically look for and welcome any exception to and disadvantage of believing an assertion. Here each honestly and courageously searches for exceptions, since even one exception can invalidate the assertion.

7. While there seems nothing wrong in having a strong interest in being right, there should be no interest in "being right at all costs." The "costs" include holding one's partner's position in contempt, using judgmentalism to attack one's partner's statements, and using controlling tactics to dominate the discussion.

It is important for partners to preface the dialogue by determining what kind of debate the partners want. They may do so by asking the following questions:

1. "About this topic, is your mind open or closed?"
2. "Would you be willing to take a provisional attitude toward this topic?"
3. "Do either of us have any emotional stuff about this topic? Are we willing to process the emotional material to clear a space for a rational discussion?"

Anthetic Conversation Analysis

Frequently people establish a pattern of conversing with each other in an automatic fashion, rarely reflecting on what they have been saying. Such conversations produce little closeness, and over time, an LVR. In order to produce more closeness, the element of reflection must be added.

In HVRs, analysis of the partners' conversations may occur from time to time. For example, partners say, "Let's analyze the way we've been talking. What do you like about it, and what do you dislike about it?" Following are additional questions partners may use in doing this kind of analysis:

1. Were you satisfied with the depth of our conversation or would you have liked more depth?
2. Was I responsive enough? Or did you feel ignored?
3. Was there any negativity?
4. Was there any self-centeredness?
5. Did I present statements provisionally?
6. Was there anything I said that you didn't like?
7. What did you like about the conversation?

Anthetic Relationship Analysis

Not only can partners analyze their conversations; they can also analyze their relationship. Partners will thereby conduct their relationship in a conscious fashion. The therapist can offer the following checklist to help couples analyze their relationship in order to see it clearly and, if they wish, take steps to correct areas where needed.

1. How much can you confide in me: Hardly at all? A little? A lot?
2. Do I connect well when we talk to each other?
3. Do I ask enough Interested Questions?
4. Do I report feelings easily?
5. Do I make power differential corrections when needed?
6. Do I do Anthetic Listening?
7. Do I consistently do Researching instead of Premature Contentiousness?
8. Do I process my negativity?
9. Do I process the feedback I get?
10. Do I easily make requests?
11. Do I make effective releasing statements?
12. Do I express enough positivity?
13. Do I use Celebratory Skills?
14. Do I use Involvement Skills?
15. Do I use Retrieval and Repair Skills?
16. Do I initiate Reconciliation when needed?
17. Do I use the skills of the Anthetic Dialogue of Ideas?
18. Do I welcome Conversation Analysis?
19. Am I always willing to work on my stuff when asked?
20. Am I open to being influenced by you?
21. Do I praise you enough?
22. Do you praise me enough?
23. Do I accept praise well?
24. Did I respect you or disrespect you?
25. Did we engage in mutuality?
26. Do I give you enough love and affection?
27. Do I see to it that you are sexually satisfied?
28. Do we agree on how to raise our children?
29. Do we have a tightly focused relationship, or are others intruding too much?

Calling Each Other to Anthetic Growth

In order to support the continued growth and enhancement of each other, partners can call each other to Anthetic Growth. This means asking or reminding a partner of the value of using their relationship for the psychological growth of each. One simple skill partners can use is to say, "I want to call you and us to continued growth in our relationship. I want us to have an optimal relationship." An alternative form is to ask the question, "Can I call you to considering growth in this area?" As the therapist teaches this skill, partners include the concept of *calling* each other, that is, evoking a growth oriented attitude, process, or behavior.

Anthetic Love

One of the most important benefits the HVR bestows is love, both the ability to express love and the ability to receive love. Clinical experience indicates that if a couple's work does not lead to love, they have not yet achieved an HVR.

The term love as used in the HVR model is not reactive love, not is it infatuation. It is called anthetic love, of which there are two types. The first type of anthetic love is universal love, an unconditional love one can feel for everyone. The second type is romantic love, which someone feels only for a special person.

To explain the first kind of anthetic love, a distinction must first be made between love and caring behavior. In this model, love is not defined as behavior. It is purely a feeling; perhaps a warm feeling; perhaps a very passionate feeling.

Caring behavior, on the other hand, is defined as behavior. It consists of giving things to a person or doing things for him or her; possibly money, gifts, driving someone to a medical appointment, or cooking a meal for someone.

When clients adopt this two-part model of love and caring, based on a feeling/behavior distinction, a great deal of confusion can be clarified about the place of love in relationships. The Anthetic application of the model helps explode five dysfunctional myths about love: That love cannot be successfully commanded or requested; that love cannot be a feeling; that love equals commitment; that love requires reciprocity; and that love is merely a neurosis.

Myth #1: Love Cannot Be Successfully Commanded or Requested

This myth underlies one of the most dysfunctional relationship patterns that can drive a couple apart. The belief that love cannot be commanded is a ludicrous version of the more modest statement, "Love cannot be requested." Clinical evidence supports that love, as a feeling, is natural to everyone. However, some people have difficulty accessing it in themselves because of internal psychological blocks. Once the blocks are addressed in therapy and removed, love can emerge. In anthetic relationship therapy, love is seen as a form of energy existing as a potential inside each person. Neurophysiological research supports this perspective. Functional magnetic resonance imaging of subjects who were intensely in love revealed activation of a complex of subcortical reward and motivation systems that lead to feelings of euphoria

(Aron, et al., 2005). In many people, especially those functioning in a low-voltage manner, the energy is blocked. It follows that when blocked, the person is unable to express love. Because the person fails to use the model of the subconscious psyche, he or she concludes that love is simply not there.

However, in clinical practice, Anthetic Therapy theorists have developed ways of helping people discover what is blocking the flow of love, whereupon it can emerge into consciousness and be felt and expressed. Once the blocks are removed, the person can easily feel and choose to express love upon request and even upon demand.

Consider the case of Myra and Ken. Myra asked Ken, "Do you love me?" Ken's answer was, "Of course I love you. Didn't I buy you a new car? I got you our wonderful house. I gave you a diamond bracelet. In fact, I give you anything you want. I'm a good provider. I take you on expensive vacations."

Hearing Ken's responses, Myra thought, "Well, that sounds right, so what am I complaining about? Why am I so dissatisfied?"

In their anthetic couple therapy sessions it took Myra a while to realize that when he talked about love, what her husband meant was material things. What she wanted, however, was affection and expressions of love. She wanted closeness and emotional intimacy and high-voltage relating. Ken, however, was afraid to give these things because of his psychological blocks. He gave material objects, because they were easy for him to give. Myra realized she was starved for love. She, in fact, said in therapy that she was considering leaving Ken if she could not get love from him.

With the help of his therapist, Ken was able to see that his problem began in childhood, where he had learned that affection was dangerous. His father had been an army officer, who demanded toughness from his sons. Ken became crystallized in the Tough polarity of functioning, and he applied that style to his marriage. When Ken saw that this low-voltage learning would lead to the breakup of his marriage, he made a conscious decision to embark on a process of converting to high-voltage relating.

As he began the process, he stated, "I don't feel love for Myra. I like her. I'm even fond of her, but I don't have any loving feelings." He viewed this state of mind as a terminal trait. However, it became apparent that he was blocked from his own source of love. Through Anthetic Dialogue, he identified a number of shoulds to avoid being soft, weak, and "wimpy." He learned releasing statements to challenge these Inner Critic injunctions. As he became freer from constriction he had developed over a lifetime of obeying shoulds against tenderness, he began to enjoy Tender polar type function. He also became more in touch with his neediness, which had also been submerged. The neediness gradually led him to contact his feelings of passionate love. He first felt some fear at the emergence of these feelings but began to see that his Inner Critic had been "protecting" him from losing himself in neediness and being overwhelmed by love, which he perceived as dangerous. He was able to make a value shift, choosing closeness over distancing. "Who needs that kind of 'protection?" he declared. "Not me anymore. All these years, I really wanted closeness and didn't know it."

He finally learned the skills of closeness and achieved flexibility in being able to deploy either Toughness or Tenderness whenever he wished. His marriage was saved, as was his relationship with his 12-year old son, who felt loved and supported by his father for the first time, and whose grades in school improved. Ken exhibits how love can be requested, and through psychological work on oneself, can be accessed and expressed.

Myth #2: Love Cannot Be a Feeling

Once again neurophysiological research challenges this myth. In research using MRI scans of people in love, Aron, et al. (2005), found that subjects' brains activated dopamine-rich portions of the brain. Their results help to explain the psychological and emotional indices of love found in previous research; specifically, euphoria, emotional dependency on and craving for emotional union with the beloved, and cathexis of the one who is loved (Fisher, 1998; Gonzaga, Keltner, Londahl, & Smith, 2001; Harris & Christenfeld, 1996; Hatfield & Sprecher, 1986; Hatfield, Schmitz, Cornelius, Rapson, 1988; Shaver, Schwartz, Kirson, & O'Connor, 1987; Tennov, 1979).

Myth #3: Love Equals Commitment

This myth holds that to love someone is to be committed to that person. When love is seen as a feeling, it is apparent that one can feel the warm feelings of love for a passing person (e.g., a baby in a stroller in a shopping center) with no commitment to care for the person implied. In addition, a person can feel warm feelings for a former partner, even though they are divorced and no resumption of commitment is desired.

One important distinction is worth drawing here. high-voltage commitment holds a special meaning; that is, that partners are willing to work on problems instead of hoping the problems will go away or simply stating, "Let's just start over." Instead, they employ the methods of intrapersonal and interpersonal skills offered in the HVR model.

Myth #4: Love Requires Reciprocity

When love is defined as a feeling, it becomes apparent that anyone can love others unconditionally, regardless of whether they return love or not. Reciprocity is no longer a condition of love. In fact, love simply feels good to the person holding it. In Anthetic Relationship Therapy, couples learn the concept of *one-way love*, that is, love that a person expresses because it feels good, whether any love is given back or not. While love that is reciprocated is rewarding, love that expects no reciprocity is an antidote to love that is given as a commodity, expecting return.

Myth #5: Love is Merely Neurosis

While it has become fashionable for some mental health professionals to declare, "Love is a disease, from which we must recover," Anthetic Relationship Therapy maintains that love is not a defect. Rather it is a spiritual energy that creates vitality and builds strong relationships. In the HVR, it is a life force.

People who cannot access love may feel depressed (termed anaclitic depression by Blatt, 1974) because when this basic life force is blocked, pleasure is decreased, devitalizing the person. Partners who cannot access love exhibit decreased intimacy, devitalization, and greater conflict (Kouneski & Olson, 2004).

THE TRAPS OF REACTIVE LOVING

Couples seeking therapy often hold a number of confused beliefs about love. An essential distinction must be made in the mind of the couple therapist, that is, distinguishing Reactive Love from Anthetic Love, so that the couple's confusion can be demystified and therapy made more efficacious. Clinical experience indicates that such confusion arises out of a number of traps into which couples fall in regard to reactive loving.

The Trading Trap

It is common for a romantic partner to say, "I love you," and to expect the partner to respond by saying, "I love you too." This ritual often becomes disconnected from real feeling. Anthetic Therapy holds that this ritual often comes from a should. The statement "I love you" can thus be a request for a trade. If the trade fails, and the partner does not reciprocate by saying "I love you too," the originating partner feels gypped and angry.

In contrast, Anthetic love does not require a trade. Because a partner feels and expresses it for herself or himself, no feeling of being gypped occurs. Were a partner to say "I love you," and the other partner say "Well, I don't love *you*," the original partner can feel and say, "Well, I still love you anyway."

In clinical experience, couples introduced to one-way love were surprised to discover that loving someone without expecting reciprocation actually felt good. The good feelings can be understood psychodynamically as an expression of the Loving Self guided by the Executive Self. Regarding the experience of one-way love, one client reported, "I radiate my warmth like the sun, because it feels good. You don't have to do anything in return. So I can love almost anyone I choose."

The "If You Loved Me" Trap

This trap is perhaps one of the most frequently reported misconceptions about love, engendering a great deal of couple conflict. An example occurs when one partner says, "If you loved me, you'd take out the garbage." In this case, the partner is confusing love with caring behavior. Once the love/caring distinction is explained to couples, they can now see that a fusion of concepts was being employed. The other partner can now say, "Yes, I love you, but I don't want to take out the garbage. The two things are separate. Let's negotiate." Now the couple is free to negotiate chores in a new way. In addition, the partners can explore the probability that the initiating partner is expressing a desire for an expression of love or affection, symbolized in the request for taking out the garbage.

The Proximity Trap

Proximity means being physically near someone, perhaps in the same city, the same house, or the same bed. Love, caring behavior, and commitment can be held from a distance. Proximity is separate from each. Moreover, a person can love someone from a distance because of a decision against proximity. The person may say, "I love you, but I don't want to be around you because of your addiction." By making this releasing statement, the person avoids the proximity trap, that is, the belief that loving someone implies spending time with them, living with them, or even maintaining contact with them.

The Low-Voltage Trap

Reactive love leads to a standard relationship characterized by two important principles: (1) avoid upsetting one's partner by honest communication and (2) avoid upsetting one's partner by making requests. Partners who aspire to high-voltage relating yet who follow these principles become trapped in an LVR.

The Trap of Sacrificial Love

A review of these reconceptualizations of love reveals that love, when seen as feelings, cannot become a sacrifice. It is a feeling, not a commodity. A person can express it and once expressed, the person does not have less of it. When love is referred to as sacrificial, confusion has occurred between love and caring. Caring can indeed become a sacrifice, in which a person denies him or herself something in order to give caring.

The True Love Trap

Clients often ask, "Is true love the right goal in choosing a life partner?" Implicit in this is a second question, "Is true love sufficient as a criterion for a successful relationship?" The answer to both is a resounding No. In fact, for a high-voltage person, it is all too easy to fall in love with a low-voltage person, thus creating a voltage mismatch. True love can easily become a trap, because it may feel genuine, yet may actually represent a conversion replay, in which one subconsciously chooses a cool, distant partner in order to convert them into a warm, loving parent.

Instead of having true love as the guiding goal, Anthetic Relationship Therapy recommends that a person seeking a partner should look first for "true High-Voltage Friendship." Employing the high-voltage profile as described throughout this book equips the searcher to differentiate a partner whose compatibility will be high. As the high-voltage friendship blossoms, and as both partners practice high-voltage skills, they create a subculture of positivity within which anthetic love can emerge.

A therapist working with an individual whose focus is partner choice can guide the person in the following sequence:

1. Qualify potential partners: Does he or she meet the high-voltage criteria?
2. If the answer is Yes, begin with high-voltage friendship.
3. If the high-voltage friendship works, it will have the possibility of evolving into high-voltage love.

ANTHETIC LOVE AND SEXUALITY

Anthetic romantic love is characterized by a softening of partners' hearts toward each other, a melting of Tough defenses, and ecstatic feelings in both. high-voltage couples in therapy have reported a number of discoveries they have made about love and sexuality.

First, they report that there is a synergistic effect between anthetic romantic love and sexuality. Such love seems to naturally evoke sexual feelings. Similarly, sexual feelings seem to naturally elicit deep feelings of love. If sex and love are sharply compartmentalized, however, this synergy does not happen. When this lack of synergy occurs, the therapist may help the couple search for psychological blocks operating to prevent the free flow of energy, then dismantle the blocks through Anthetic Dialogue.

Second, couples report that love seems to come from a spiritual (i.e., transcendent) source. Anthetic Therapy holds that if one sees God as the source of love, partners can open to that source and channel the love through themselves to each other and to others.

Third, sexuality also seems to come from a spiritual source. When infused with spiritual rapture and ecstasy, sheer lust has the ability to transform and empower anthetic romantic love. Sex without anthetic love, on the other hand, seems simply a biological release.

Fourth, sexual behavior can occur in almost any romantic relationship, but couples report that it best occurs when in the context of love, nonjudgmental acceptance, caring behavior, involvement, and the commitment that marriage brings, that is, in the context of high voltage.

Fifth, couples have found that sex is much more ecstatic if accompanied by verbal expressions of love, in fact, profuse expressions.

Of course, it is obvious that a person can love another, engage in caring behavior, be involved, and have closeness without any sexual intimacy at all, because the relationship is non-romantic.

LOVE AND THE EXPRESSION OF LOVE

Still another important distinction must be made in the reconceptualization of love, that is, the distinction between simply experiencing love for someone and in expressing that feeling to the person. Expressions of love include a loving touch or hug or saying the words "I love you" or "I have loving feelings for you."

A person may love another without necessarily doing anything about it or expressing it in any way. For example, a female teacher who especially loves one of her male students may choose not to express it, not only because it might be misinterpreted, but also because it would have a negative effect on the target person. In other words, just because one feels love does not mean he or she has to express it.

CARING BEHAVIOR: IS IT BACKED BY SHOULDS OR BY LOVE?

Caring behavior can be motivated either by Inner Critic shoulds or by Anthetic love. It is best if motivated by love. If motivated by shoulds, it may demand reciprocity and set up failed trades. For example, Janna and Cody told the therapist about an unresolved argument. Janna said, "I've gone with Cody to Sunday dinner at his family's every week. Now, the one time I ask him to go with me to my niece's first birthday party, he says he doesn't want to come. I'm furious that after all I've done, he won't do this one little thing for me." Janna's anger indicates that her caring behavior in going to Sunday dinners had been motivated at least partially by shoulds with the hope of reciprocity. Cody admitted he knew nothing about her expectations that he would also attend her family functions. The couple had never talked about their desires and expectations in this area. Janna's trading was tacit. She stated, "He should have automatically wanted to come with me."

Focused Relating

In romantic relationships, high-voltage commitment also includes having a tightly focused coupling. For example, it includes having an exclusive sexual relationship; partners putting each other first; making decisions mutually; and giving up old attachments, especially to former romantic relationships.

Love and Merging

Love in the HVR usually results in a certain amount of merging, in which a new definition of self as a shared identity occurs. Partners see themselves as a We-self, rather than as mere individuals. This idea has been validated empirically in the self-expansion research of A. Aron and his colleagues (Aron & Aron, 1997; Aron, A., Aron, E.N., & Smollan, 1992). Their research found that close couples' self concepts expand to include the other.

One danger may occur in which merging may be so crystallized that one loses oneself in one's partner. What this means is that one partner continually defers excessively to the other for the sake of being loved. In order to avoid this problem, couples learn in Anthetic Relationship Therapy to be able to disengage at any time, and then merge at any time. The key concept here is Anthetic Orthogonal Flexibility.

Multiple Bonds

HVRs are usually characterized by multiple bonds. In addition to love, sex, and familial bonds, they share interest in personal growth, along with other companionship bonds through such interests as dancing, literature, art, music, history, sports, and so on. The more bonds, the more satisfying and stable the relationship.

Love that Lasts

Because of its psychological infrastructure, Anthetic love is love that lasts. It is marked by partners' championing of each other's growth. It results in a mutually enhancing relationship.

ANTHETIC LOVE AND PROFOUND LOVE

As mentioned, Anthetic love is one-way love; love that is given without a demand for reciprocity. Although one-way love feels good for the lover to give, one more step is possible: Profound Love. This love occurs when each partner expresses Anthetic love to the other. At this point, love goes both ways, but in such a way that each love is not contingent on the other. In other words, each person engages in one-way love. Clients in couple therapy who have achieve Profound Love report that it produces the most blissful relationship they have ever experienced.

High-Voltage Romantic Love

When applied to romantic relationships, high-voltage principles can provide the most intense closeness. Following is a test to determine whether a person values the intensity of high-voltage romantic love.

Do You Want High-Voltage Romantic Love?

Directions: Circle each of the following letters T or F for True or False, as it applies to you.

1. When we go out walking, I like to hold hands, even in public places. **T F**
2. I want a lot of touching in my relationship. **T F**
3. When my partner and I go on vacation, I want us to go to the same place together. **T F**
4. I like to have frequent sexual experiences with my partner. **T F**
5. I am physically attracted to my partner. **T F**
6. I like to talk about romantic times we've had in the past. **T F**
7. I like to tell my partner "I love you" several times a day, whether or not my partner reciprocates by saying "I love you too." **T F**
8. I like it when my partner says "I love you." **T F**
9. I like to spend a lot of time with my partner; I like to do things with my partner as often as possible. **T F**
10. I like to take baths or showers with my partner. **T F**

11. I like to massage and be massaged by my partner. **T F**
12. I like melting in my partner's embrace. **T F**

Scoring: Add up the number of T items you checked. The more items checked, the greater your desire for a romantic HVR. You might also ask your partner to take this test so you can compare scores. If there is no romantic HVR currently in your life, you can use this test to screen a possible candidate for one.

PSYCHOLOGICAL BLOCKS TO LOVE

The Anthetic Relationship Therapy position is that one's core personality, the Natural Self, wants to give and receive Anthetic love and closeness. This holds true unless the person has psychological blocks to doing so. Following are a number of blocks identified in partners in couple counseling:

- Fear of Being Hurt Again: The individual sees closeness as dangerous, although the only symptom may be reluctance to becoming deeply involved with anyone. The cause of such reluctance identified in individuals with this block is an Inner Child figure that has been hurt in the past and fears further rejection and hurt, thus fearing all intimacy.
- Fear of Being Known: The person has fear of disclosing himself or herself to others. This fear has its roots in Inner Critic functioning, in which the emotional punishment of defectiveness is prominent. Once a person learns Anthetic Inner Critic challenging, this fear can be dismantled so the person no longer relies on rigid defenses.
- Fear of Losing Autonomy: This fear appears in some Tender Dependent persons who have a history of sacrificing autonomy in close relationships in order to receive emotional supplies of love and approval. In an attempt to defend against further loss of self, the person may revert to a Self-Sufficient stance as a reaction to a former Dependent way of life. Anthetic Relationship Therapy focuses on helping the person be close and still free. The process involves both Inner Critic challenging of conceptual fusions (for example, "Just because I say 'I love you' doesn't mean I have to comply with your requests") as well as Inner Figure work with defensive figures (for example, the Protector).
- Fear of Losing Individuality: For persons with a powerful need for love, craving love may lead them to abandon their individuality for it. Anthetic Relationship Therapy assists partners in supporting each other's individuality. One skill couples learn is, "Are you selling out right now? Because I don't want you to."

- Fear of Being Taken Advantage of: Because the Anthetic approach holds love as simply a feeling and not caretaking, loving does not entail being taken advantage of. The therapist assists clients with this fear by teaching them to use releasing statements such as, "Just because I express my love doesn't mean I have to do what my partner wants. I can be loving and say No. I can be loving and protect myself in any way I choose. I have the right to make decisions based on what's in my best interest. I'm not here to live up to their expectations."
- Anger, Hatred, and Vindictiveness: Acting out these three feelings, along with other forms of negativity, is guaranteed to block the person's feelings of love from flowing freely.
- Self-Centeredness: When a person is unable to see others in an empathic way, loving them becomes difficulty.
- Seeing Love as Weakness: Those who see love as weakening will do their best to live by Inner Critic shoulds to be strong. They will adopt the Tough polarity. They may say, as did one business executive in couple counseling, "I don't care whether other people like me, as long as they fear me and respect me." With this attitude, the person will not have the right to be soft and tender in a relationship, because his or her Inner Critic denies that right. The therapist can assist partners with this problem by helping them challenge the Inner Critic and the powerful prototypes that were the source of that injunction. In addition, therapy can include reframing expressing affectionate love not as weakness but as a courageous thing to do; in fact, a symbol of strength.

LOVE AS OPENING THE HEART; LOVE AS SOFTENING THE HEART

Once partners have chosen to value high-voltage relating and have learned skills for such relating, love requires an open heart and a soft heart. Unfortunately, negativity in partners often has become a default mode that proposes to protect them by defending them against giving and receiving love. In this process, partners harden their hearts. They end up seeing their partners as "bad."

In order to have a heart soft enough to express and accept love, more than a simple decision is required. Valuing having a soft heart is step one; working on opening and softening is step two. Such work follows a three step process, utilizing the intrapersonal and interpersonal skills outlined in this book. First, work on reducing or eliminating negativity. Second, work on accessing and processing fears. Third, work on accessing and expressing positive feelings.

CONCLUDING COMMENTS

Anthetic Relationship Therapy holds that in every person is a basic goodness, even though it becomes barnacled over with reactivity. Although the voice of negativity may be strong, the voice of love can become even stronger.

The HVR model proposes that in order to have optimal relationships, partners must be patient with each other; must be empathic toward each other's feelings. They must sensitively respond to each other's feedback, offering caring, valuing, and love despite flaws and weaknesses.

As more and more people use the values, principles and skills of this model, the possibility increases of creating relationships that are loving safe havens from a reactive society, not battlegrounds to play out old animosities carried over as ghosts from childhood. These safe havens can provide sanctuaries in which partners may expand their horizons and pursue their dreams rather than worry about what other people will think of them, how they can win at all costs, or how they can get revenge.

Each partner must choose between reactivity and love. Each must choose whether to be part of the problem, as enablers or accomplices, or part of the solution.

The Anthetic model appears to offer a new archetype for the positive relationships people seek. One of its strengths is its scope: it applies not just to marriage but to all relationships. Another strength is its psychological infrastructure, which leads to specific methods for working toward emotional closeness, beyond simple exhortations to be close. A third strength is that, like any scientific endeavor, it is always open to change as new learnings occur.

The technology is now available. The path is now clear for this new model, Anthetic love, to inform the lives of everyone. If all goes well, the result in the future will be a culture of positivity throughout the world, within which HVRs can emerge everywhere and become as common then as reactive relationships are today.

References

Acevedo, B.P., & Aron, A. (2009). Does a long term relationship kill romantic love? *Review of General Psychology, 13,* 59–65.

Adams, G., Anderson, S.L., & Adonu, J.K. (2004). The cultural grounding of closeness and intimacy, In D.J. Mashek, & A. Aron (Eds.), *Handbook of closeness and intimacy* (pp. 61–78). Mahwah, NJ: Lawrence Erlbaum Associates.

Agnew, C.R., Loving, T.J., Le, B., & Goodfriend, W. (2004). Thinking close: Measuring relational closeness as perceived self-other inclusion. In D.J. Mashek, & A. Aron (Eds.), *Handbook of closeness and intimacy* (pp. 103–115). Mahway, NJ: Lawrence Erlbaum Associates.

Ainsworth, M.D.S., Blehar, M.C., Waters, E., & Wall, S. (1978). *Patterns of attachment: A psychological study of the strange situation.* Hillsdale, NJ: Lawrence Erlbaum Associates.

Aron, A., & Aron, E. (1997). Self-expansion motivation and including other in the self. In S. Duck (Ed.), *Handbook of personal relationships* (2nd ed., pp. 251–270). New York: Wiley.

Aron, A., & Aron, E.N. (1986). *Love as an expansion of self: Understanding attraction and satisfaction.* New York: Hemisphere.

Aron, A., Aron, E.N., & Norman, C. (2001). The self-expansion model of motivation and cognition in close relationships and beyond. In M. Clark, & G. Fletcher (Eds.), *Blackwell Handbook of Social Psychology, Vol. 2: Interpersonal Processes* (pp. 478–501). Oxford, England: Blackwell.

Aron, A., Aron, E.N., & Smollan, D. (1992). Inclusion of other in the self scale and the structure of interpersonal closeness. *Journal of Personality and Social Psychology, 63,* 596–612.

Aron, A., Fisher H., Mashek, D.J., Strong, G., Haifang, L., & Brown, L.L. (2005). Reward, motivation, and emotion systems associated with early-stage intense romantic love. *Journal of Neurophysiology, 94,* 327–337.

Aron, A.P., & Mashek, D.J. (2004). Conclusion, In D.J. Mashek, & A. Aron (Eds.), *Handbook of closeness and intimacy* (pp. 415–428). Mahway, NJ: Lawrence Erlbaum Associates.

Aron, A.P., Mashek, D.J., & Aron, E.N. (2004). Closeness as including other in the self. In D.J. Mashek, & A. Aron (Eds.), *Handbook of Closeness and Intimacy* (pp. 27–41). Mahwah, NJ: Lawrence Erlbaum Associates.

Arriaga, X.B., Goodfriend, W., & Lohmann, A. (2004). Beyond the individual: Concomitants of closeness in the social and physical environment. In D.J. Mashek, & A. Aron (Eds.), *Handbook of Closeness and Intimacy* (pp. 287–303). Mahwah, NJ: Lawrence Erlbaum Associates.

Assagioli, R. (1965). *Psychosynthesis.* New York: Hobbs, Dorman.

Baldwin, M.W. (1992). Relational schemas and the processing of social information. *Psychological Bulletin, 112,* 461–484.

Baldwin, M.W., Keelan, J.P.R., Fehr, B., Enns, V., & Koh-Rangarajoo, E. (1996). Social-cognitive conceptualization of attachment working models: Availability and accessibility effects. *Journal of Personality and Social Psychology, 71,* 94–109.

Baucom, D.H., Epstein, N., Rankin, L.A., & Burnett, C.K. (1996). Assessing relationship standards: The Inventory of Specific Relationship Standards. *Journal of Marriage and the Family, 10,* 72–88.

Baumeister, R.F., & Leary, M.R. (1995). The need to belong: Desire for interpersonal attachments as a fundamental human motivation. *Psychological Bulletin, 117,* 497–529.

Becker, J.V., & Skinner, L.J. (1983). Assessment and treatment of rape-related sexual dysfunctions. *Clinical Psychologist, 36,* 102–105.

Berley, R.S., & Jacobson, N.S. (1984). Causal attributions in intimate relationships: Toward a model of behavioral marital therapy. In P. Kendall (Ed.), *Advances in cognitive-behavioral research and therapy: Vol. 3.* (pp. 2–90). New York: Academic Press.

Berne, E. (1961). *Transactional analysis in psychotherapy.* New York: Grove Press.

Berne, E. (1972). *What do you say after you say hello?* New York: Grove Press.

Berns, S.B., Jacobson, N.S., & Gottman, J.M. (1999). Demand-withdraw interaction in couples with a violent husband. *Journal of Consulting and Clinical Psychology, 67,* 666–674.

Berscheid, E., Snyder, M., & Omato, A.M. (2004). Measuring closeness: The Relationship Closeness Inventory (RCI) revisited. In D.J. Mashek, & A. Aron (Eds.), *Handbook of Closeness and Intimacy* (pp. 81–101). Mahwah, NJ: Lawrence Erlbaum Associates.

Blatt, S.J. (1974). Levels of object representation in anaclitic and introjective depression. *The Psychoanalytic Study of the Child, 29,* 107–157.

Bloom, B., Asher, S., & White, S. (1978). Marital disruption as a stressor: A review and analysis. *Psychological Bulletin, 85,* 867–894.

Bowlby, J. (1982). *Attachment and loss: Vol. 1. Attachment.* New York: Basic. (Original work published 1969).

Bowlby, J. (1988). *A secure base.* New York: Basic Books.

Brennan, K.A., & Shaver, P.R. (1995). Dimensions of adult attachment, affect regulation, and romantic relationship functioning. *Personality and Social Psychology Bulletin, 21,* 267–283.

Briere, J. (1992). *Child abuse trauma: Theory and treatment of the lasting effects.* Newbury Park, CA: Sage.

Burman, B., & Margolin, G. (1992). Analysis of the association between marital relationships and health problems: An interactional perspective. *Psychological Bulletin, 112,* 39–63.

Christensen, A. (1987). Detection of conflict patterns in couples. In K. Hahlweg, & M.J. Goldstein (Eds.), *Understanding major mental disorder: The contribution of family interaction research* (pp. 250–265). New York: Family Process Press.

Christensen, A. (1988). Dysfunctional interaction patterns in couples. In P. Noller, & M.A. Fitzpatrick (Eds.), *Perspectives on marital interaction* (pp. 31–52). Avon, England: Multilingual Matters.

Christensen, A., & Heavey, C.L. (1990). Gender and social structure in the demand/withdraw pattern of marital conflict. *Journal of Personality and Social Psychology, 59,* 73–81.

Christensen, A., & Heavey, C.L. (1993). Gender differences in marital conflict: The demand/withdraw interaction pattern. In S. Oskamp, & M. Costanzo (Eds.), *Gender issues in contemporary society* (pp. 113–141). Newbury Park, CA: Sage.

Collins, N.L. (1996). Working models of attachment: Implications for explanation, emotion, and behavior. *Journal of Personality and Social Psychology, 71,* 810–832.

Collins, N.L., & Feeney, B.C. (2000). A safe haven: An attachment theory perspective on support seeking and caregiving in intimate relationships. *Journal of Personality and Social Psychology, 78,* 1053–1073.

Collins, N.S., & Read, S.J. (1990). Adult attachment, working models, and relationship quality in dating couples. *Journal of Personality and Social Psychology, 58,* 644–663.

Corey, G. (1991). *Theory and practice of counseling and psychotherapy* (4th ed.). Pacific Grove, CA: Brooks/Cole.

Cosmides, L., & Tooby, J. (1992). Cognitive adaptations for social exchange. In J.H. Barkow, L. Cosmides, & J. Tooby (Eds.), *The adapted mind: Evolutionary psychology and the generation of culture* (pp. 163–228). New York: Oxford University Press.

Crossley, N. (1996). *Intersubjectivity: The fabric of social becoming.* London: Sage.

Dew, J., & Wilcox, W.B. (2013). Generosity and the maintenance of marital quality. *Journal of Marriage and Family, 75,* 1218–1228.

Doss, B.D., Simpson, L.E., & Christensen, A. (2004). Why do couples seek marital therapy? *Professional Psychology, 35,* 608–614.

Duck, S. (Ed.). (1997). *Handbook of personal relationships: Theory, research and interventions* (2nd ed.). New York: Wiley.

Dusay, J. (1977). *Egograms: How I see you and you see me.* New York: Harper & Row.

Earley, J. (2012). *Activating your inner champion instead of your inner critic.* Larkspur, CA: Pattern Systems Books.

Earley, J., & Weiss, B. (2010). *Self-therapy for your inner critic: Transforming self-criticism into self-confidence.* Larkspur, CA: Pattern Systems Books.

Edelstein, R.S., & Shaver, P.R. (2004). Avoidant attachment: Exploration of an oxymoron. In D.J. Mashek, & A. Aron, *Handbook of closeness and intimacy* (pp. 397–412). Mahway, NJ: Lawrence Erlbaum Associates.

Elliott, J.E. (1991). Defusing conceptual fusions: The 'just because' technique. *Journal of Cognitive Psychotherapy, 5,* 227–229.

Elliott, J.E. (1992a). Compensatory buffers, depression, and irrational beliefs. *Journal of Cognitive Psychotherapy, 6,* 175–184.

Elliott, J.E. (1992b). Use of anthetic dialogue in eliciting and challenging dysfunctional beliefs. *Journal of Cognitive Psychotherapy, 6,* 137–143.

Elliott, J.E. (1994). Using releasing statements to challenge shoulds. *Journal of Cognitive Psychotherapy, 7,* 291–296.

Elliott, J., & Elliott, K. (1997). Philosophical counseling as an aspect of anthetic therapy. Paper presented at American Society of Philosophical Counselors & Psychotherapists World Conference. New York.

Elliott, J., & Elliott, K. (2000). *Disarming Your Inner Critic.* Lafayette, LA: Anthetics Institute Press.

Elliott, K. (2006). Anthetic inner critic work as a method for relapse prevention: Identifying and overcoming self-critical beliefs. *Alcoholism Treatment Quarterly, 24,* 109–119.

Elliott, K., & Elliott, J. (2010). *Establishing criteria for a life partner, friend, or relative.* Lafayette, LA: Anthetics Institute Press.

Elliott, K., & Elliott, J. (2013). *The theory and practice of anthetic group therapy.* Lafayette, LA: Anthetics Institute Press.

Elliott, K., & Elliott, J. (2014). *Hearts entwined: The love letters of therapist-soulmates.* Lafayette, LA: Anthetics Institute Press.

Elliott, K.J. (1995). The WILFY method: Unlearning lessons from the past. *Journal of Cognitive Psychotherapy, 9,* 259–266.

Elliott, K.J. (1999). The "inner critic" as a key element in working with adults who have experienced childhood sexual abuse. *Bulletin of the Menninger Clinic, 63,* 240–253.

Epstein, S. (1994). Integration of the cognitive and psychodynamic unconscious. *American Psychologist, 49,* 709–724.

Epstein, N.B., & Baucom, D.H. (2002). *Enhanced cognitive-behavioral therapy for couples: A contextual approach.* Washington, DC: American Psychological Association.

Fairbairn, W.R.D. (1952). *Psychoanalytic studies of the personality.* London: Tavistock.

Feeney, B.C., & Collins, N.L. (2001). Predictors of caregiving in adult intimate relationships: An attachment theoretical perspective. *Journal of Personality and Social Psychology, 80,* 972–994.

Feeney, J.A. (1998). Adult attachment and relationship-centered anxiety: Responses to physical and emotional distancing. In J.A. Simpson, & W.S. Rholes (Eds.),

Attachment theory and close relationships (pp. 189–218). New York, NY: Guilford Press.

Feeney, J.A. (1999). Adult romantic attachment and couple relationships. In J. Cassidy, & P.R. Shaver (Eds.), *Handbook of attachment: Theory, research, and clinical applications* (pp. 355–377). New York: Guilford Press.

Feeney, J.A., & Noller, P. (1990). Attachment style as a predictor of adult romantic relationships. *Journal of Personality and Social Psychology, 58*, 281–291.

Fehr, B. (2004). A prototype model of intimacy interactions in same-sex friendships. In D.J. Mashek, & A. Aron (Eds.), *Handbook of closeness and intimacy* (pp. 9–26). Mahwah, NJ: Lawrence Erlbaum Associates.

Feinauer, L.L., & Stuart, D.A. (1996). Blame and resilience in women sexually abused as children. *American Journal of Family Therapy, 24,* 31–40.

Finkelhor, D., & Browne, A. (1985). The traumatic impact of child sexual abuse: A conceptualization. *American Journal of Orthopsychiatry, 55,* 530–541.

Firestone, R.W., & Catlett, J. (1999). *Fear of intimacy.* Washington, DC: American Psychological Association.

Firestone, R.W., & Firestone, L. (2004). Methods for overcoming the fear of intimacy. In D.J. Mashek, & A. Aron (Eds.), *Handbook of closeness and intimacy* (pp. 375–395). Mahwah, NJ: Lawrence Erlbaum Associates.

Fisher, H.E. (1998). Lust, attraction, and attachment in mammalian reproduction. *Human Nature, 9,* 23–52.

Fletcher, G.J.O., & Clark, M.S. (Eds.). (2000) *Blackwell handbook of social psychology: Interpersonal processes.* Oxford, England: Blackwell.

Fraley, C., & Shaver, P. (1998). Airport separations: A naturalistic study of adult attachment dynamics in separating couples. *Journal of Personality and Social Psychology, 75,* 1198–1212.

Frank, E., & Stewart, B.D. (1984). Depressive symptoms in rape victims. *Journal of Affective Disorders, 1,* 269–277.

Freud, S. (1900/1955). *The interpretation of dreams.* New York: Basic Books.

Freud, S., (1914/1949). On narcissism: An introduction. *The international psychoanalytic library,* vol. 4. London: The Hogarth Press.

Freud, S. (1915/1957). The unconscious. *The international psycho-analytic library,* vol.14. London: The Hogarth Press.

Freud, S. (1923). The ego and the id. *The international psychoanalytic library,* Vol. 12. London: The Hogarth Press, 1949.

Gazzaniga, M. (1985). *The social brain.* New York: Basic Books.

Geoff, T., Fletcher, G.J.O., & Lange, C. (1997). On-line empathic accuracy in marital interaction. *Journal of Personality and Social Psychology, 72,* 839–850.

Geselbracht, R. (2004). National Archives February 2004 Feature: The Love Story of Harry and Bess Truman. Retrieved 2/28/2015 from http://www.archives.gov/calendar/features/2004/02.html

Gigy, L., & Kelly, J.B. (1992). Reasons for divorce: Perspectives of divorcing men and women. *Journal of Divorce and Remarriage, 18,* 169–187.

Gonzaga, G.C., Keltner, D., Londahl, E.A., & Smith, M.D. (2001). Love and the commitment problem in romantic relations and friendship. *Journal of Personality and Social Psychology, 81,* 247–262.

Gottman, J.M. (1993). The roles of conflict engagement, escalation, and avoidance in marital interaction: A longitudinal view of five types of couples. *Journal of Consulting and Clinical Psychology, 61,* 6–15.

Gottman, J.M. (1994). *What predicts divorce?* Hillsdale, NJ: Lawrence Erlbaum Associates.

Gottman, J.M. (1999). *The marriage clinic: A scientifically based marital therapy.* New York: W.W. Norton.

Gottman, J.M., Coan, J., Carrere, S., & Swanson, C. (1998). Predicting marital happiness and stability from newlywed interactions. *Journal of Marriage and the Family, 60,* 5–22.

Green, E.J., Elliott, K., & Myrick, A.C. (2014). Deepening couples counseling through inner critic dialogue: A case study. *The Family Journal: 22: 2,* 156–161.

Greenberg, L.S., & Johnson, S.M. (1988). *Emotionally focused therapy for couples.* New York: Guilford.

Greenberg, L., Safran, J., & Rice, I. (1989). Experiential therapy: Its relation to cognitive therapy. In A. Freeman, K. Simon, L. Beutler, & H. Arkowitz (Eds.), *Comprehensive handbook of cognitive therapy* (pp. 169–187). New York: Plenum Press.

Gunthrip H. (1971). *Psychoanalytic theory, therapy and the self.* New York: Basic Books.

Harris, C.R., & Christenfeld, N. (1996). Gender, jealousy, and reason. *Psychological Science, 7,* 364–366.

Hatfield, E., Schmitz, E., Cornelius, J., & Rapson, R.L. (1988). Passionate love: How early does it begin? *Journal of the Psychology of Human Sexuality, 1,* 35–51.

Hatfield, E., & Sprecher, S. (1986). Measuring passionate love in intimate relationships. *Journal of Adolescence, 9,* 383–410.

Hazan, C., & Shaver, P. (1987). Romantic love conceptualized as an attachment process. *Journal of Personality and Social Psychology, 52,* 511–524.

Heidegger, M. (1962). *Being and time.* San Francisco: Harper.

Horney, K. (1950). *Neurosis and human growth.* New York: Norton.

Husserl, E. (1960). *Cartesian meditations.* The Hague: Nijhoff.

Ickes, W. (1997). *Empathic accuracy.* New York: Guilford.

Ickes, W., & Simpson, J.A. (1997). Managing empathic accuracy in close relationships. In W. Ickes (Ed.), *Empathic accuracy* (pp. 218–250). New York: Guilford.

Ickes, W., Hutchison, J., and Mashek, D. (2004). Closeness as intersubjectivity: Social absorption and social individuation. In D. Mashek, & A. Aron (Eds.), *Handbook of closeness and intimacy* (pp. 357–373). Mahwah, NJ: Lawrence Erlbaum Associates.

Ickes, W., Stinson, L., Bissonnette, V., & Garcia, S. (1990). Naturalistic social cognition: Empathic accuracy in mixed-sex dyads. *Journal of Personality and Social Psychology, 39,* 730–742.

Ito, T.A., Larsen, J.T., Smith, N.K., & Cacioppo, J.T. (1998). Negative information weighs more heavily on the brain: The negativity bias evaluative categories. *Journal of Personality and Social Psychology, 75,* 887–900.

Jankowiak, W.R., & Fischer, E.F. (1992). A cross-cultural perspective on romantic love. *Ethnology, 31,* 149–155.

Johnson, S.M. (1996). *The practice of emotionally-focused marital therapy: Creating connection.* New York: Brunner/Mazel.

Johnson, S. (2004). *The practice of emotionally focused couple therapy: Creating connections.* New York: Brunner/Rutledge

Johnson, S.M., & Greenberg, L.S. (1994). Emotion in intimate relations. In S.M. Johnson, & L.S. Greenberg (Eds.), *The heart of the matter: Perspectives on emotion in marital therapy.* (pp. 3–22). New York: Brunner/Mazel.

Jung, C.G. (1956). *Two essays on analytical psychology.* New York: Meridian.

Jung, C.G. (1961). *Memories, dreams, reflections.* New York: Vintage.

Jung, C.G. (1968). *Analytical psychology: Its theory and practice—The Tavistock lectures.* London: Routledge and Kegan Paul. (Original work published 1935).

Kant, I. (1900). *Critique of pure reason.* New York: Co-operative Publication Society.

Kelley, H.H. (1979). *Personal relationships: Their structures and processes.* Hillsdale, NJ: Lawrence Erlbaum Associates.

Kelley, H.H. (1997). The "stimulus field" for interpersonal phenomena: The source of language and thought about interpersonal events. *Personality and Social Psychology Review, 1,* 140–169.

Kelley, H.H., Berscheid, E., Christensen, A., Harvey, J.H., Huston, T.L., Levinger, G., et al. (Eds.). (1983). *Close relationships.* New York: Freeman.

Kirkpatrick, L.A., & Davis, K.E. (1994). Attachment style, gender, and relationship stability: A longitudinal analysis. *Journal of Personality and Social Psychology, 66,* 502–512.

Kirkpatrick, L.A., & Hazan, C. (1994). Attachment styles and close relationships: A four-year prospective study. *Personal Relationships, 1,* 123–142.

Klein, M. (1948). *Contributions to psychoanalysis.* London: Hogarth Press.

Kouneski, E.F. (2002). *Five types of marriage based on ENRICH: Linking intrapersonal and interpersonal characteristics.* Unpublished doctoral dissertation, University of Minnesota, Twin Cities.

Kouneski, E.F., & Olson, D.H. (2004). A practical look at intimacy: ENRICH couple typology. In A. Aron, & D.J. Mashek (Eds.), *Handbook of closeness and intimacy* (pp. 117–133). Mahwah, NJ: Lawrence Erlbaum Associates.

Kris, E. (1952). *Psychoanalytic explorations in art.* New York: International Universities Press.

Kugel, J. (2010). An inner relationship focusing approach to transforming the inner critic. Dissertation abstracts international: Section B. *The sciences and engineering, 71,* 33–59.

Laurenceau, J., Rivera, L.M., Schaffer, A.R., & Pietromonaco, P.R. (2004). Intimacy as an interpersonal process: Current status and future directions. In D.J. Mashek, & A. Aron (Eds.), *Handbook of closeness and intimacy* (pp. 61–78). Mahwah, NJ: Lawrence Erlbaum Associates.

Lederer, W.J., & Jackson, D.D. (1968). *The mirages of marriage.* New York: W.W. Norton.

Levenson, R.W., & Ruef, A.M. (1992). Empathy: A physiological substrate. *Journal of Personality and Social Psychology, 63,* 234–246.

Levy, K.N., Blatt, S.J., & Shaver, P.R. (1998). Attachment styles and parental representations. *Journal of Personality and Social Psychology, 74,* 407–419.
Lindberg, F.H., & Distad, L.J. (1985). Post-traumatic stress disorders in women who experienced childhood incest. *Child Abuse and Neglect, 9,* 329–334.
Linehan, M.M. (1987). Dialectical behavior therapy for borderline personality disorder. *Bulletin of the Menninger Clinic, 51,* 261–276.
Low, A.A. (1950). *Mental health through will-training.* Boston: The Christopher Publishing House.
Lussier, Y., Sabourin, S., & Turgeon, C. (1997). Coping strategies as moderators of the relationship between attachment and marital adjustment. *Journal of Social and Personal Relationships, 14,* 777–791.
Markus, H., & Nurius, P. (1987). Possible selves: The interface between motivation and the self-concept. In K. Yardley, & T. Honess (Eds.), *Self and identity: Psychosocial perspectives.* Chichester, England: Wiley.
Mashek, D.J., & Aron, A.P. (2004). Introduction. In A. Aron, & D.J. Mashek (Eds.), *Handbook of closeness and intimacy* (pp. 1–9). Mahwah, NJ: Lawrence Erlbaum Associates.
Mashek, D.J., & Sherman, M.D. (2004). Desiring less closeness with intimate others. In D.J. Mashek, & A. Aron, *Handbook of closeness and intimacy* (pp. 343–356). Mahwah, NJ: Lawrence Erlbaum Associates.
Mehl, M.R., Vazire, S., Holleran, S.E., & Clark, C.S. (2010). Eavesdropping on happiness: Well-being is related to having less small talk and more substantive conversations. *Psychological Science, 42,* 1537–1546.
Mikulincer, M., Gillath, O., Halevy, V., Avihhou, N., Avidan, S., & Eshkoli, N. (2001). Attachment theory and reactions to others' needs: Evidence that activation of the sense of attachment security promotes empathic responses. *Journal of Personality and Social Psychology, 81,* 1205–1224.
Mikulincer, M., & Shaver, P.R. (2001). Attachment theory and intergroup bias: Evidence that priming the secure base schema attenuates negative reactions to outgroups. *Journal of Personality and Social Psychology, 81,* 97–115.
Myers, D.G., & Diener, E. (1995). Who is happy? *Psychological Science, 6,* 10–19.
Olson, D.H., & Olson, A.K. (1999). PREPARE/ENRICH program: Version 2000. In R. Berger, & M.T. Hannah (Eds.), *Preventive approaches in couples therapy.* Philadelphia: Brunner/Mazell.
Paul, L. (1970). The cruel inner critic. *Psychotherapy, Theory, Research and Practice, 7,* 178–180.
Perls, F.S. (1969). *Gestalt therapy verbatim.* Lafayette, CA: Real People Press.
Prager, K.J. (2000). Intimacy in personal relationships. In S. Hendrick and C. Hendrick (Eds.), *Close relationships* (pp. 229–244). Thousand Oaks, CA: Sage.
Prager, K.J., & Roberts, L.J. (2004). Deep intimate connection: Self and intimacy in couple relationships. In D.J. Mashek, & A. Aron (Eds.), *Handbook of Closeness and Intimacy* (pp. 43–60). Mahwah, NJ: Lawrence Erlbaum Associates.
Reis, H.T., Clark, M.S., & Holmes, J.G. (2004). Perceived partner responsiveness as an organizing construct in the study of intimacy and closeness. In D.J. Mashek, & A. Aron (Eds.), *Handbook of closeness and intimacy* (pp. 201–225). Mahway, NJ: Lawrence Erlbaum Associates.

Resick, P.A., & Schnicke, M.K. (1992). Cognitive processing therapy for sexual assault victims. *Journal of Consulting and Clinical Psychology, 60,* 748–756.

Roberts, L.J., & Greenberg, D.R. (2002). Observational windows to intimacy processes in marriage. In P. Noller, & J. Feeny (Eds.), *Understanding marriage: Developments in the study of couple interaction. Advances in Personal Relationships Series* (pp. 118–149). Cambridge, MA: Cambridge University Press.

Rook, K.S. (1987). Social support versus companionship: Effects on life stress, loneliness, and evaluations by others. *Journal of Personality and Social Psychology, 52,* 1132–1147.

Rothbard, J.C., & Shaver, P.R. (1994). Continuity of attachment across the life span. In M.B. Sperling, & W.H. Berman (Eds.), *Attachment in adults: Clinical and developmental perspectives* (pp. 31–71). New York: Guilford Press.

Rusbult, C.E., Kumashiro, M., Coolsen, M.K., & Kirchner, J.L. (2004). Interdependence, closeness, and relationships. In D.J. Mashek, & A. Aron (Eds.) *Handbook of closeness and intimacy* (pp. 137–161). Mahwah, NJ: Lawrence Erlbaum Associates.

Rusbult, C.E., Kumashiro, M, Stocker, S.L., Kirchner, J.L., Finkel, E.J., & Coolsen, M.K. (2005). Self processes in interdependent relationships: Partner affirmation and the Michelangelo phenomenon. *Interaction Studies, 6,* 375–391.

Ryff, C.D. (1989). Happiness is everything, or is it? Explorations on the meaning of psychological well-being. *Journal of Personality and Social Psychology, 57,* 1069–1081.

Sanderson, C.A. (2004). The link between the pursuit of intimacy goals and satisfaction in close relationships: An examination of the underlying processes. In D.J. Mashek, & A. Aron (Eds.), *Handbook of closeness and intimacy* (pp. 247–266). Mahwah, NJ: Lawrence Erlbaum Associates.

Sartre, J. (1956). *Being and nothingness.* New York: Philosophical Library.

Satir, V. (1964). *Conjoint family therapy.* Palo Alto, CA: Science and Behavior Books.

Satir, V. (1972). *Peoplemaking.* Palo Alto, CA: Science & Behavior Books.

Satir, V. (1978). *Your many faces.* Berkeley, CA: Celestial Arts.

Schafer, R. (1960). The loving and beloved superego in Freud's structural theory. *The Psychoanalytic Study of the Child, 15,* 163–188.

Scharff, D.E., & Scharff, J.S. (1987). *Object relations family therapy.* Northvale, NJ: Aronson.

Scharff, D.E., & Scharff, J.D. (1991). *Object relations couple therapy.* Northvale, NJ: Aronson.

Schwartz, R.C. (1995). Internal family systems therapy. New York: Guilford Press.

Shaver, P., Schwartz, J., Kirson, D., & O'Connor, C. (1987). Emotion knowledge: Further exploration of a prototype approach. *Journal of Personality and Social Psychology, 52,* 1061–1086.

Simpson, J.A., Rholes, W.S., & Nelligan, J.S. (1992). Support seeking and support giving within couples in an anxiety-provoking situation: The role of attachment styles. *Jounal of Personality and Social Psychology, 62,* 434–446.

Simpson, J.A., Rholes, W.S., & Phillips, D. (1996). Conflict in close relationships: An attachment perspective. *Journal of Personality and Social Psychology, 71,* 899–914.

Stinckens, N., Lietaer, G., & Leijssen, M. (2013). Working with the inner critic: Process features and pathways to change. *Person-Centered & Experiential Psychotherapies, 12,* 59–78.

Sweeney, M., Ziskind, E., & Schwartz, R. (Eds.). (2013). Internal family systems therapy: New dimensions. New York: Taylor & Francis.

Tennov, D. (1979). *Love and limerance: The experience of being in love in new york.* New York: Stein and Day.

Vohs, K.D., & Baumeister, R.F. (2004). Sexual passion, intimacy, and gender. In D.J. Mashek, & A. Aron (Eds.) *Handbook of closeness and intimacy* (pp. 189–199). Mahwah, NJ: Lawrence Erlbaum Associates.

Vorhaus, P. (1966). Spotting and stopping the inner saboteur. *Psychoanalytic Review, 53,* 451–459.

Watzlawick, P., Beavin, J.H., & Jackson, D.D. (1967). *Pragmatics of human communication: A study of interactional patterns.* New York: W.W. Norton.

Westerlund, E. (1992). *Women's sexuality after childhood incest.* New York: Norton.

Wile, D.B. (1992). *Couples therapy: A nontraditional approach.* New York: Wiley.

Index

About the Authors

James Elliott, Ph.D., is the creator of Anthetic Therapy and Anthetic Relationship Therapy. He is the author with Kathryn Elliott of *Disarming Your Inner Critic* and *Hearts Entwined: The Love Letters of Therapist-Soulmates.* He founded Anthetics Institute in Berkeley, California and in Lafayette, Louisiana.

Kathryn Elliott, Ph.D., LPC-S, LMFT, is Director of Anthetic Therapy Center and retired Associate Professor of Counselor Education.

James and Kathryn presented at numerous professional conferences including American Psychology Association, American Association for Marriage and Family Therapy, and American Association of Sex Educators, Counselors, and Therapists. They have published numerous articles in professional journals including *The Family Journal, Bulletin of the Menninger Clinic, Journal of Cognitive Psychotherapy, Journal of Mental Health Counseling,* and *Alcoholism Treatment Quarterly.* Kathryn and James lived their own High-Voltage Relationship for twenty-two years until James's death in 2011.

www.ingramcontent.com/pod-product-compliance
Ingram Content Group UK Ltd.
Pitfield, Milton Keynes, MK11 3LW, UK
UKHW012038150926
475560UK00001B/79

9 781442 238107